Liquid Herbal Drops In Everyday Use

3rd Edition

Daniel J. Gagnon
Medical Herbalist

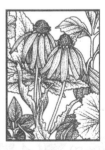

Botanical Research and Education Institute
Santa Fe, New Mexico

Please note!
This book is designed to provide you with some herbal care
options. Bear in mind that the herbs listed in this book are
for prevention and for problems that do not require major
medical intervention. This book is not intended to replace
the expertise of a primary care physician. If the complaint
you are treating is not getting better, or if it is getting
worse, consult a doctor.

Author: Daniel J. Gagnon
Editor: Jerilynn J. Blum
Editorial Assistant: DorothyAnn Collom
Publishing Consultant: JoEllen Bokar
Editorial Consultants: JoEllen Bokar, Charlotte Des Roches,
                         Jamie Reagan
Graphic Design & Layout: John Cole
Book & Cover Illustrations: Angela Werneke
  (© 1995 Angela Werneke)

Publisher: Botanical Research & Education Institute, Inc.
                 2442 Cerrillos Road, Suite 296
                 Santa Fe, NM 87501

♻ *Post consumer recycled paper*

About Daniel J. Gagnon

Daniel has been a practicing herbalist since 1976. Born in French Canada, he relocated to Santa Fe, New Mexico in 1979. There he furthered his studies in medical herbalism, pharmacognosy and related subjects at the Santa Fe College of Natural Medicine, the College of Santa Fe and the College of Pharmacy at the University of New Mexico.

His passion for helping others was born out of his own childhood health problems. His experience with conventional medical treatment of eczema, asthma and allergies motivated him to seek gentler, more soothing healing modalities, which ultimately put him on the path to becoming an herbalist. His goal is to educate both the public and the medical profession about the practical, healing applications of herbal medicine.

Daniel is frequently called upon as an herbal consultant by medical doctors, naturopaths, chiropractors and acupuncturists. He is the co-author of *Breathe Free*, a nutritional and herbal care book for the respiratory system; and the author of *Healing Herbs for the Nervous System*. He regularly teaches seminars and college credit classes on herbal therapeutics, both in the United States and in Canada.

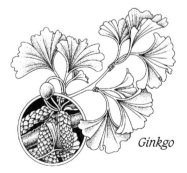

Ginkgo

Table of Contents

Author's Introduction:
About This Book

September 1997, Third Edition

Dear Herbal Enthusiast,

My goal in writing *Liquid Herbal Drops in Everyday Use*—whether you are just beginning to learn about herbs or whether you are already knowledgeable—is to provide you with the best, most practical, easy-reference guide to herbal medicine in the marketplace today.

There are many books that generally detail "which herbs are good for what." What this book does differently is help you to focus, in practical and specific terms, on *which* herbs to take at *what* times and *how* best to take them.

It has been thrilling to receive so much positive feedback on the first and second editions of this book. I never expected that over 70,000 copies would be sold in a little under four years!

Thank you to all the readers who wrote to say how useful the book was to them. I also appreciate the readers who wrote to ask specific herbal questions that were not answered in the first edition.

Last year, we incorporated many new features in the second edition that were suggested by readers, as well as friends, fellow retailers

WERNEKE © 1995

Calendula

6

and health professionals. We greatly expanded the number of Questions and Answers. The **Herbal Repertory** grew to include 22 new single extracts and formulas. The Health Condition Index, over a third longer, was expanded to list 371 different health conditions responsive to herbal treatment. Seven new easy-reference tables addressing common health problems were added to the book. Most of all, we worked diligently to keep the price of this book low so that more people can benefit from this valuable knowledge.

This year, the third edition has been updated to feature a different binding and to index more health conditions in the Health Condition Index. This index is still definitely one of the most complete indexes of its kind for any size book.

The formulas listed in this book are ones that I have put together over the past ten years. I recommend them in my practice as a medical herbalist and also in my role as a consultant to professional health practitioners.

All the formulas listed have been tested and improved upon as a result of ongoing scientific testing and/or client feedback; and all have been proven safe and effective. All are available at natural food markets, herb stores and natural pharmacies throughout the United States and Canada.

I welcome any of your suggestions or comments on how this book can be improved for the next edition. I also want to hear about your ideas on which additional herbs should be included next time.

I hope you enjoy reading this book. May it enlighten you with helpful insights and point the way in your quest for health.

Herbally Yours,

Daniel J. Gagnon

Chapter 1:
The Ten Elements of Good Health

As a human being, you are a physical, mental, emotional and spiritual ecosystem...

It is important to understand that good physical health does not exist independently of the lifestyle decisions we make. We each exist in a personal and collective ecosystem where our physical bodies interrelate with our internal processes and our external surroundings. No system of health care, herbal or otherwise, can "cure" a physical condition existing in an ecosystem that is out of balance.

Personal choice is the most important element in maintaining the health of your ecosystem. Who we are is the sum of the choices that we make every day. We constantly choose what to eat and drink, who to be with, what to talk about, which movies to watch, and so forth. All of these choices may seem insignificant when we make them one by one. But when we add them together, they have a tremendous impact on our bodies. For example, going to a fast food place occasionally does not have major health consequences. But when fast food becomes our main food supply, our bodies become overloaded with fats, sodium and free radicals; and starved for fiber, vitamins and minerals. Over a period of time, this type of diet leads to degenerative diseases. It may take years, but it will happen. Each choice that we make either adds up to "health" in the positive column or "health distress" in the negative column.

Maintaining our ecosystem is a dynamic process. It is a little bit like being on a see-

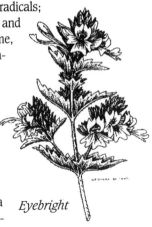

Eyebright

saw. As we move away from our "center," our energy is sapped so that we are more subject to extreme highs and lows. Conversely, the sooner we take measures to stay close to our pivot point of balance, the less energy we need to expend to stay healthy. This "surplus" energy can then be used for doing things in our lives that give us joy, happiness and contentment.

If you wish to optimize your health, minimize your health risks and increase your resilience, or if you are confronted with a health problem, I suggest you examine how balanced you are in the following ten areas. Do you need to modify or delete elements that are out of balance in your life? What choices are you making in these ten areas?

In many ways, health is incredibly easy to maintain. It doesn't require detailed scientific or medical knowledge. Balancing these ten elements on a daily basis will lead you to good health and help keep you there.

1. EXERCISE Are you exercising?

Exercise at least five times a week for one half hour. One of the best forms of exercise is walking because it is low impact and inexpensive! It can be practiced by virtually anyone at almost any time and its benefits start accruing immediately. All you need is a good pair of walking shoes.

2. REST Are you getting enough rest?

Set aside some time every day just to do nothing except relax and breathe, even if it is only for 15 minutes. Place a priority on getting enough restful sleep. You can't repair your body and your soul without enough rest.

3. NUTRITION Is your diet fully supporting your body?

Are you eating whole foods and organic foods? Refined, highly-processed foods and foods treated with pesticides during the growing process present problems to your "ecological system," ranging from not providing the nutrients your body needs to the possibility of causing disease. "Organic" foods are not treated with pesticides, nor do they contain harmful preservatives. Eating a wide variety of preferably organic whole grains, vegetables and fruits will improve your physical functioning. Include at least one portion a day of the following green leafy vegetables: Swiss and red chard, kale, collards, brussel sprouts, parsley, mustard greens, turnip greens, chicory greens, dandelion or beet greens, spinach, cabbage, watercress, purslane, okra, broccoli, or any sprouts, including alfalfa, sunflower and soybean. *Are you taking your supplements?* Vitamins and minerals are helpful in supplementing your diet/metabolism, even if you are eating organic foods. Taking a full spectrum vitamin/mineral supplement every day is a must. *Do you drink sufficient water?* Drink 64 ounces of water a day to stay fully hydrated. *And, don't forget your herbs!*

4. NATURE Do you spend time outdoors?

Nothing can replace being with the natural elements when it comes to balancing your Self. Devoting time weekly to getting some fresh air and sun is critical to the overall health of your personal ecosystem.

5. CREATIVITY Do you have some sort of creative outlet that keeps you active?

Creative outlets can range from work to that hobby you never seem to have time for. Staying active and in contact with the rest of the world is integral to good health.

6. EMOTIONAL BALANCE Are you emotionally healthy?

Do you have repetitive episodes of anger, fear or grief that keep you out of balance? There is nothing wrong with having feelings. They give us valuable information about what we may need to change in our lives to be happier. Emotional imbalance becomes an issue when feelings are either repressed or allowed to irrationally rule us. If either of these extremes is true for you, have you taken measures to identify and change your emotional patterns? You can choose to cultivate joy and a sense of humor to nourish your ecosystem.

7. GOALS Are you mentally stimulated?

To thrive, everyone should have something—whether it's doing volunteer work, spearheading a project, or working toward a goal—that demands brain activity. We all need direction and purpose in life.

8. MUTUAL SUPPORT Are you giving and receiving love in your life?

Having a loving and accepting support system is critical to

healing. Ecosystems, by their very nature, are dependent upon relationship. Giving and getting support and love from your family, friends, or support group is essential to good health.

9. FAITH Do you regularly communicate with your Higher Self or your Higher Power?

Many a wise soul has said that we must feel connected to a higher power to feel balanced and fulfilled in life. In keeping with your personal belief system, do you make time for this aspect of yourself or for spiritual guidance to help you in your daily life?

10. CHOICE Do you take personal responsibility for your life?

A critical step in your self-creation of a healthy body and a healthy life involves taking responsibility for your actions. At any given moment, we have choice. Taking personal responsibility is the key that unlocks the door to integrating and balancing all of the other elements of healthy living discussed above.

Maximize what herbs can do for you...

Herbs truly have the ability to assist you in making significant shifts in both chronic and acute physical conditions. You can further maximize the healing effects of herbs by bringing yourself into a more complete state of balance suggested by the elements above. Is there anything missing in your life? What does your personal ecosystem need? Remember that the choices you make daily give you the power to shape your life!

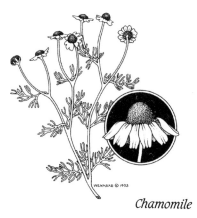

Chamomile

11

Chapter 2:
Understanding Herbal Medicine

Q: What is herbal medicine and who uses it?

Sometimes called botanical medicine or phytotherapy, herbal medicine is the use of herbs for health purposes. Herbs have been used by mankind for thousands of years. According to the World Health Organization, eighty percent of the world's population still depends on herbal medicine as a primary way of healing. Thousands of herbs are recognized worldwide for their health benefits. In the last twenty five years, the United States has been going through a major rediscovery of medicinal herbs. During this time, Traditional Chinese Medicine, Ayurvedic medicine from India, and South American herbs have also been quickly entering the American herbal tradition.

Q: How does herbal medicine interface with current medical practices?

Herbal medicine for some is a total alternative to orthodox allopathic medical treatments. For others, herbal medicine stands alongside conventional medicine as another choice, depending on the health issue at hand.

Overall, herbal medicine offers prevention, affordability, and safety. Many people see herbal medicine as an alternative to drugs or surgery, which are the treatment modalities most often used in allopathic medicine when health problems reach a crisis point. Drugs very often have serious side effects and their costs can be prohibitive. In some instances the drugs that are given to patients are more dangerous than the diseases they are intended to treat. The perspective of herbal medicine is that orthodox allopathic medicine is geared to crisis management, where the majority of the time people go to the doctor when their problems have escalated to the point that they require drastic measures, such as drugs or surgery. Oftentimes the drugs are too strong or the surgery is too drastic for the problem at hand, but in the orthodox system these are the major treatment choices.

Enter Herbal Medicine. Herbs are attractive because they are affordable and because they optimize a person's ability to deal with health problems that may not need drugs or surgery, but may still prevent people from fully enjoying life. Health problems of this nature include conditions such as eczema, emphysema and endometriosis. Herbs generally assist the healing process by helping rebuild and strengthen weak organ systems, causing many nagging health problems to disappear. In the field of holistic medicine, herbs are not taken to "cure" disease but instead are used as tools to help rebalance and support the body in its quest for health.

Q: Specifically, what do herbs offer me in the way of health care benefits?

Herbs offer you eight benefits:

1. Simplicity and accessibility: Good quality herbs are now readily available in almost every conceivable delivery system, i.e. capsules, tablets, tea bags, liquid herbal extracts, loose herbs, lozenges and salves. Most forms of herbs are available at local natural products stores and natural pharmacies.

2. Safety: All of the herbs explored in this book are safe. In the few instances where a pre-existing condition may limit the use of herbs, specific contraindications have been noted for those herbs. In some cases, if the use of a large amount of an herb may cause side effects, these have been noted also. Remember that any substance can have a side effect if enough of it is ingested. For example, eating too many prunes may lead one to discover the laxative effect of these fruits. *The bottom line is that herbs are safe but you must, as with any medication, heed dosage directions and any contraindications or side effects noted.*

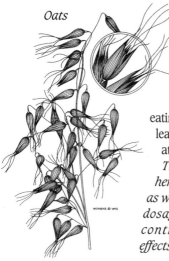

Oats

13

3. Tolerance: Most people do very well with herbs. Sometimes conventional drugs have adverse side effects that can only be offset by additional drugs. Herbs, on the other hand, do not cause such a domino effect, as they are generally easily absorbed and assimiliated by the body.

4. Effectiveness: Herbs with gentle actions are usually not recognized by "experts" as having any therapeutic benefits. But anybody who has taken a cup of chamomile tea for sleep problems will attest to the fact that you don't need to be hit over the head with a drug-like effect in order to enjoy the benefits of herbs. Herbs are effective despite the fact that they cannot be "tested" in the same manner as drugs. Part of the reason that the effects of herbs are not as well documented as drugs is that herbs do not contain just one single active principle. This makes it challenging for scientists to devise experiments to study herbs, but herbs are proven and effective healing agents, nevertheless.

5. Economy: Many herbs offer the same benefits as drugs for a fraction of what drugs cost. For example, Proscar™ costs the average man suffering from benign prostatic hypertrophy (swollen prostate) approximately $2.50 a day for treatment. The same problem can be addressed with the herb Saw Palmetto for about 50 cents a day.

6. Empowerment: Herbs allow you, personally, to do something for your health, at the precise time you need to do it.

7. Ecology for your "ecosystem": Herbs are substances that your body can work with. They are not foreign substances. They ellicit a positive response from the body, aiding it to return to a balanced state.

8. Environmental friendliness: When herbs are certified organically-grown or are ethically wildcrafted, their harvesting has very little or no negative impact on the planet. The pharmaceutical industry, on the other hand, manufactures drugs using complex and environmentally negative petroleum by-products and other chemicals.

Q: How do herbs differ from drugs in the way they interact with the body?
There is a fundamental difference between how conventional drugs and herbs interrelate with the body. One

works within the body for a limited time period. The other trains the body for the future.

Antibiotics bypass the immune system to kill intruders; therefore, they do not teach the body how to defend itself in the future. Antibiotics also disrupt the ecology of the body and permit other microorganisms to grow and take over the normal flora in the intestines, as well as in other locations in the body. Drugs leave toxic residues that the body must either detoxify or store somewhere in the body.

On the other hand, herbs holistically help re-educate the body to heal itself. For example, Echinacea will stimulate your immune system not only to fight a current infection, but also to recognize intruders a lot more rapidly and to respond a lot more aggressively the next time your body encounters the same bug. Because herbs are less toxic and leave no hard-to-deal-with residues, the body regains its full balance much more easily. None of the herbs addressed in this book leave behind hard-to-deal-with residues in the body.

Metaphorically, drugs give a man a fish and feed him for a day. Herbs teach a man how to fish so that he can feed himself for a lifetime.

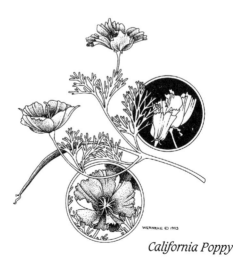

California Poppy

Chapter 3:
Choosing Which Herbs Are Best for You

Q: What forms do herbs come in?
Basically there are two categories of herbs—fresh herbs and dried herbs. Dried herbs can be found whole, in pieces, or powdered. Herbal capsules, tablets, and 99 percent of herbal syrups and tea bags are made from dried herbs. Herbal salves and liquid herbal extracts can be made from both dried and fresh herbs. Herbs that are still fresh, before drying, can only be made into fresh teas or liquid herbal extracts (also called tinctures).

Q: What are liquid herbal extracts?
Liquid herbal extracts are herbs that have been processed in such a way that the active ingredients are suspended in a liquid medium, usually alcohol and water.

Q: How are liquid herbal extracts made?
Liquid herbal extracts are produced by subjecting herbs, in ground or powdered form, to precise ratios of water and alcohol for specified lengths of time in order to capture the active ingredients of those herbs. In my opinion, two methods yield the most potent extracts. Fresh herbs are most potent when they are "kinetically macerated." Using this method, herbs are first agitated in an alcohol and water solution for 12 hours, and then soaked in that same liquid solution for a minimum of two weeks. For dried herbs, the active ingredients are best extracted with the use of a special glass funnel called a "percolator." Using this method, an alcohol and water solution

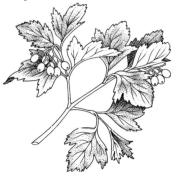

Cramp Bark

is poured over dried herbs packed in the percolator, and the resulting liquid herbal extract slowly drips from the percolator. Notice in both methods that no heat is used, since heat is very damaging to the potency of the herbs' active ingredients.

Q: Why do you focus on herbs in liquid herbal extract form instead of herbs in capsule or tablet form?

The success of herbal products as healing agents is dependent upon how active their ingredients are when you ingest them. For maximum therapeutic benefits, therefore, it is very important to take herbs in the form that best captures and preserves their active ingredients. In my opinion, liquid herbal extracts offer, by far, the most therapeutically beneficial form of herbs available on the market today.

Herbal tablets contain fillers, binders and other materials necessary to the process of compressing ground herbs into tablet form. In addition, the body has to dissolve tablets before it can begin to assimilate the herbs. Herbal capsules are better than tablets because they do not contain the extra manufacturing materials and they dissolve easily in the stomach. However, if the body is not digesting and assimilating well, the potential therapeutic benefits of herbs in capsule form diminishes. Also keep in mind that many herbs in tablet or capsule form are ground months prior to appearing on store shelves. They lose many of their active ingredients through evaporation and oxidation both during the grinding process and while in storage.

Herbs in extract form, on the other hand, contain no fillers, binders, or "extra" ingredients, and they are immediately assimilated into the body. Nothing has to be broken down or digested in order for the body to absorb them. The process of extraction removes the active ingredients from the fresh or dried herbs and puts them into a solution that preserves them. In this liquid form, the herbs are immediately available for assimilation into the bloodstream, glands and organs. Even a person with poor digestion and assimilation can enjoy maximum benefits from liquid herbal extracts.

Q: Is it better to buy liquid herbal extracts made from fresh herbs or dried herbs?

There is no simple answer to this question. I believe it depends on your therapeutic objectives, i.e. why you are taking the herbs you are taking. Nettle, for example, can be used fresh or dried. As an agent to increase mineral absorption, dried Nettle offers the most benefits. On the other hand, fresh Nettle will offer optimum hay fever relief because once Nettle is dried, its hay fever-alleviating properties disappear. Certain herbs, such as Blue Cohosh, Dong Quai, Golden Seal and Milk Thistle, are better used dried because the drying process modifies and enhances their medicinal action. Other herbs, such as Chamomile, Oat Seeds, Peppermint and Shepherd's Purse, should be processed while fresh in order to preserve their delicate volatile oils and other fragile constituents.

Whether you choose fresh herbs or dried herbs depends on each herb's specific constituents and the therapeutic goal you are trying to achieve. Therefore, some liquid herbal extracts are made from fresh herbs and others are made from dried herbs. In some formulas, fresh and dried forms are blended together. This assures that you get the best form of each herb for the specific problems you are addressing.

Q: Why is alcohol used to make liquid herbal extracts?

There are three main reasons alcohol is used. First, alcohol and water are used to make liquid extracts because both of these substances are necessary to insure full extraction of all the active ingredients of the herbs. Golden Seal best illustrates this principle. Boiling this root for hours in water will extract its water soluble properties but will fail to extract its main anti-inflammatory property, called hydrastine. It takes a minimum of 60 percent alcohol to extract this constituent.

Second, alcohol assists in the absorption of the herb by the body's mucous membranes. Third, alcohol acts as a natural preservative, preventing contamination and assuring a longer shelf life.

The alcohol content in different extracts ranges from as little as 20 percent to as high as 95 percent, because the amount of alcohol required for maximum extraction is dependent upon the properties of the herbs. Vinegar and glycerin do not succeed in replacing alcohol as efficient extractive agents.

Q: When the label says an extract has 70 percent alcohol in it, does that mean the remaining 30 percent is herbs and water?

No it doesn't. 100 percent of the mixture in the bottle contains herbs. To use an analogy, let's say you stir one tablespoon of sugar into four ounces of water. You still have four ounces of water, but it is now sweet. The sugar is contained within the water but is no longer visible as a separate ingredient. The water is now permeated with sugar. It is the same with herbs. If a particular extract uses 70 percent alcohol and 30 percent water to extract and preserve the herbs, both the 70 percent alcohol and the 30 percent water are imbued with herbs. They hold the herbs just as the water in this analogy holds the sugar.

Q: As a recovering alcoholic, should I avoid herbal extracts containing alcohol?

Based on the information given here, I believe that extracts containing alcohol have a very low capability of physiologically re-addicting a person. But because the psychological aspect of addiction is so important, I also encourage you to follow your beliefs if you think taking extracts containing alcohol would be a problem for you.

In a nutshell, here is how alcohol in liquid herbal extracts compares to alcoholic beverages. Ingesting 40 drops of an extract containing 70 percent alcohol, three times a day for ten days, is the same as drinking one beer over the course of ten days. Furthermore, putting each extract dosage in hot water to evaporate the alcohol before taking it would make the bottle of beer in this analogy last for 30 days. Another analogy that puts the alcohol content of the average extract dosage in perspective is to look at the amount of alcohol in a banana. Eating one ripe banana provides more alcohol in your diet than does one full dosage of an extract. This is

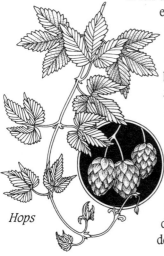

Hops

why some people have used herbal extracts successfully even while they were in the process of stopping drinking. There is even one herb, called Kudzu, that aids in suppressing alcohol cravings.

Q: What is the difference between liquid herbal extracts that are made with alcohol and extracts that are alcohol-free?

The herbs in liquid herbal extracts made with alcohol are generally stronger. They have more active ingredients available to the user and they last longer. Unfortunately, alcohol-free extracts have very few active ingredients and, as such, they are not a good value for the money.

One study I was involved with compared alcohol-free extracts of Golden Seal to alcohol-containing extracts of Golden Seal by measuring the levels of two major active alkaloids. The study verified that there is a direct correlation between alcohol percentage and the level of alkaloids present. The lower the alcohol, the lower the healing alkaloids. The alcohol-free extracts tested were so low in potency that they were practically useless. According to the study's ratings, you would need ten bottles of the alcohol-free extracts rated "best" and 256 (yes, that is 256) bottles of the alcohol-free extracts rated "worst" to equal one good bottle of alcohol-based extract. Based on this study, I feel that the alcohol-free extracts currently available on the market are a waste of time and money.

Q: I have read that I should buy herbs that are "standardized." What is standardization?

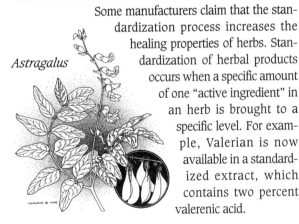

Astragalus

Some manufacturers claim that the standardization process increases the healing properties of herbs. Standardization of herbal products occurs when a specific amount of one "active ingredient" in an herb is brought to a specific level. For example, Valerian is now available in a standardized extract, which contains two percent valerenic acid.

In the last few years there has been a tremendous push in the herb industry to "standardize" herbal products primarily because of two strong influences. First, medical doctors are being drawn to herbs by patients who are growing uncomfortable with synthetic drugs and who are, therefore, requesting less harsh, but equally effective natural remedies. Coming from an orthodox, pharmaceutical framework, doctors feel more comfortable when they can recommend products that have "active ingredients" found in measurable and consistent amounts. Thus they are encouraging standardization of herbs. Second, in response to pressure from medical doctors to bring herbs in line with how drugs are standardized, some herb companies are trying to develop such products.

In my opinion, standardization runs counter to the holistic view that each herb is an ecosystem that combines all of its parts to heal and balance our bodies.

Q: So, does standardization increase the healing potential of herbs?

Even though considerable debate on this subject rages on, I strongly believe that using whole herbs is superior to standardizing fragments of herbs. To support my viewpoint, I point to three issues that are outstanding in the debate over this topic.

First, it is not known exactly what the active ingredient is in 98 percent of herbs. Research on Echinacea illustrates how this question of "Which one is the active ingredient?" is still unanswered. In the late 1970s and the early 1980s, research concluded that the polysaccharides in Echinacea had many immunostimulating activities. Based on this, many European companies started standardizing their extracts to achieve a specific amount of polysaccharides. Then subsequent research revealed that alcohol soluble constituents were even more stimulating to the immune system than the polysaccharides. Key questions that came out of all this research were: "To which active ingredient should a plant be standardized?" and "Does standardizing certain ingredients in herbs make them better products?" In my opinion, this research has failed to prove that standardized ingredients are superior to whole herb extracts for most herbs.

The second issue that seems to color the perception that standardized herbs are the way to go is that success in standardization with a few herbs has been assumed to be possible for all herbs. Yes, there are a handful of standardized herbs that have been shown to be effective in certain situations. For instance, Feverfew extracted to yield 400 mcg of parthenolide is helpful for migraine headaches. Also, Milk Thistle with standardized silymarin levels of 125 mg is used for serious liver pathologies. But if you are using Milk Thistle as a liver protectant, a whole seed extract protects the liver just as well as a standardized extract, at a fraction of the cost. In addition, the whole seed contains many other innate substances that help support the healing of the liver. So the successful standardization of five or six herbs is simply not applicable to all herbs, or applicable for all their uses. Remember that in 98 percent of herbs, we do not yet know what the active ingredient is. This means that, at the present time, standardization is possible in about only two percent of herbs.

Finally, it seems to me that this debate and the practice of standardization of herbs is another instance of science trying to improve Nature by dissecting her. Research into the standardization of Valerian provides us with a pertinent example. First, it was thought that the essential oils were the active ingredients of Valerian. But when the essential oils alone were administered to people, they achieved only partial results. Then it was thought that valepotriates were the active ingredients until testing revealed only partial results again. Still later, valerenic acid was thought to be the active ingredient. More testing, same results. The irony is that each testing process actually supports the theory that the whole plant gives more complete results than any fraction of the plant.

Q: Does it matter if the herbs I take are organic?
As an herbalist concerned about our environment, I strongly recommend that herbal consumers choose certified organically-grown herbs.

First, choosing organically cultivated herbs helps lessen over-harvesting of herbs in the wild. For example, Echinacea and Golden Seal, among other herbs, are facing near extinction unless we start cultivating these plants. Second, certified organic farmers make sure they have crops year after year by not compromising their land for short-term gain. Therefore, by buying organic, you support renewing the land. Third, certified organic farmers are inspected by a third party certifying agency, insuring that they practice sustainable, chemical-free and pesticide-free farming techniques. This means that organic herbs truly support your healing as well as the health of our planet.

Q: How long do herbs in different forms retain their effectiveness?

Form	Shelf-Life
Powdered Herbs	1–6 Months
Herbal Capsules	1–6 Months
Tea Bags	1–6 Months
Herbal Tablets	2–12 Months
Whole Dried Leaves	2–12 Months
Whole Dried Roots	1–3 Years
Liquid Herbal Extracts	3–20 Years

This chart points out that the more an herb is ground or reduced in size, the more rapidly it will lose its beneficial properties. In general, whole herbs tend to retain their medicinal properties or "shelf life" longer than other forms of herbs. This chart also shows that alcohol-based liquid herbal extracts maintain a longer shelf life than other forms of herbs. Once the herbs are extracted in a liquid medium, very little evaporation, oxidation or degradation of active ingredients occurs.

Q: How should I care for liquid herbal extracts to keep them fresh?
For optimum shelf life, I suggest a three point approach. First, keep your extracts away from sunlight (away from windows). Second, keep your extracts away from extreme temperatures (do not store them in the glove compartment of your car in summer time). Third, keep bottle caps firmly closed. With alcohol-based extracts, no refrigeration is ever required. Remember that with reasonable care, your herbal extracts will last a minimum of three years and more.

Q: How can I tell if an extract has gone "bad"?
In my experience with *alcohol-based liquid extracts*, it is rare for extracts not to last for years when they are stored

correctly. The only exception to this rule that I have found is with extracts containing Ephedra (Ma Huang). If you have an extract containing Ephedra and you see that the herbs are clumping together in the bottle or on the dropper, I recommend discarding the bottle.

Q: What should I look for when I buy liquid herbal extracts?

1) Sufficient Alcohol Amount and Cold Processing: Be aware of the production process that herbs have gone through. Choose extracts with a minimum of 20 percent alcohol used to extract the complete spectrum of active ingredients from herbs. A minimum of 20 percent alcohol content also acts as a preservative and prevents contamination by fungus, bacteria and viruses. When extracts are made from whole herbs ground cryogenically (cold grinding) minutes prior to extraction, no constituents are destroyed by friction-induced heat during the grinding process. Cold process kinetic maceration for fresh herbs or cold process percolation for dried herbs yields more active ingredients in finished extracts than in herbs processed by using other methods.

2) Organically Grown Herbs: Choose herbal extracts made from certified organically grown herbs. When certified organically grown herbs are not available, choose wild harvested herbs that have been picked in the wild in regions not exposed to pesticides, herbicides or fertilizers.

3) Liquid Herbal Extracts in Formulas: Choose herbal formulas, especially when you are not quite sure which single herb(s) to choose. The formulas listed in this book have been blended, tested and approved by medical herbalist Daniel Gagnon.

Echinacea purpurea

Chapter 4:
Taking Medicinal Herbal Extracts

Q: Why choose formulas instead of single herbs?

To get the results you hope to achieve in treating your health problem, it is important to choose the right herbs. Although this book lists both single extracts and formulas, and both are effective healing agents, I generally favor formulas because I feel they offer you greater health benefits, greater affordability and greater convenience.

For example, if you look in the **Health Condition Index** of this book under arthritis, you will see that several single extracts (Devil's Claw, Feverfew or Meadowsweet for internal use and Arnica for external use) and two formulas (Arthrotonic™ and Herbaprofen™) are recommended. If you then read the description of each of the single extracts in the **Herbal Repertory** (Chapter 7), you will see that each extract offers you a choice of what herb or herbs you might elect to take to relieve your arthritis. For example, Devil's Claw works on the arthritic inflammation and helps the liver excrete waste that contributes to inflammation, Feverfew works over the long term to relieve pain, and Meadowsweet supports the kidneys to also excrete waste that aggravates inflammation. As you can see, a certain amount of detailed knowledge of the body's physiology and your particular symptomology are required to distinguish what to take.

On the other hand, when you read the description of the recommended formula Arthrotonic™, you will see that it combines Devil's Claw and nine other herbs, which all perform specific functions to relieve the symptoms of arthritis and help the body get healthy again. The formula Herbaprofen™ combines Jamaican Dogwood, Meadowsweet and seven other herbs, again all with specific functions for, in this case, relieving pain. The guesswork of determining which single extracts to take has been eliminated for you. The cost of buying one or two formulas versus buying all of the single extracts included in each formula is significantly less. The level of support for your arthritis is greatly amplified because a formula is stronger than the sum of its herbal parts. Each herb complements the others and together they form a stronger coalition to strengthen and support the body in its quest for health.

Q: Do I use herbs differently when I have an acute condition, as opposed to when I have a chronic condition?

During an **acute phase** (rapid onset, severe symptoms, short course, as in colds or flu) of a disease, it is desirable to take herbs on a frequent basis to maintain a high amount of the herbs' active constituents in the bloodstream. This way, the stimulation or sedation that the herbs offer can constantly bathe the affected tissues. If the therapeutic level falls off, the invading microorganisms or the inflammation threatening the tissues will grow. Your body then has to redouble its efforts to get back to normal. Taking care of the acute phase quickly and completely prevents the problem from becoming chronic or recurrent.

During a **chronic phase** (long duration, ongoing or recurring symptoms, as in arthritis) of a disease, it is more important to take herbs on a regular basis over a long period of time in order to offer the challenged tissues healing support. In this phase, you need to supply tissues with nutrients and pharmacologically active substances on a daily basis so that they can heal and resume their normal functioning.

Arthritis again provides us with a clear example of how herbs address acute versus chronic phases

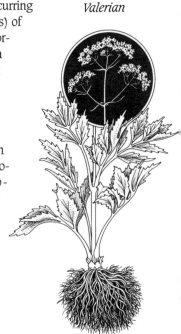

Valerian

of a disease. In the chronic phase of arthritis, a person will have stiffness and dull pain in the joints; whereas during an acute flare-up, a lot of inflammation and sharper pain, as well as swelling, will be present. Both phases have to be helped, but in a different way. In an acute flare-up, the strategy is to decrease the inflammation and get rid of the waste products that are contributing to the inflammation. This requires small, frequent dosages. During a chronic phase, the strategy is to stabilize and help repair the tissues, and prevent future flare-ups. This requires larger dosages, taken fewer times a day, over long periods of time.

Q: What is the best time of day to take liquid herbal extracts?

In most instances, I suggest taking extracts between meals, apart from food, because that is when they are more easily absorbed by the body. This way, extracts enter the bloodstream readily and immediately start the healing process. A few herbs, however, are better taken before meals. For example, bitter herbs help to tone up the stomach and increase production of hydrochloric acid and other digestive enzymes. Others, like sleep aid herbs, are better taken one hour before bedtime to permit relaxation and more restful sleep. Note the dosage notation under each herb in the **Herbal Repertory** (Chapter 7) for specific directions on timing.

Q: Is it advisable to take a particular extract, such as Echinacea, continually?

For most herbs, including Echinacea, I recommend alternating periods of herbal support with periods of rest. I call this concept "pulsing." See the general guidelines for pulsing which follow. On the other hand, some herbs are best taken for long periods of time without a break. This is why the dosage recommendations given for each herb in the **Herbal Repertory** (Chapter 7) note when herbs should be pulsed and, in some instances, exactly how they should be pulsed. If pulsing is not indicated, that means that the herb can be taken long term without pulsing.

Pulsing means that you take an herb for a certain length of time, then you take a rest from it for awhile; or you can alternate it with another herbal product for a certain length of time. The purpose of pulsing is to give your body a chance to work on its own without herbal intervention. It also seems that the body responds better to herbs when you resume taking them after a rest.

Two-thirds of herbs should be pulsed to receive the maximum benfits. One-third are best not pulsed.

I recommend two possible ways of pulsing. For herbs you are taking for *short or long* periods of time, take for five days, stop for two days, and then repeat. For herbs you are taking for *long* periods of times, take for three weeks, stop for one week, and then repeat. Please note that some of the dosages indicated in the **Herbal Repertory** (Chapter 7) recommend specific pulsing periods. If pulsing is not recommended for an herb, then that herb can be taken, or may *need* to be taken, continually for long periods of time in order to achieve results.

Q: How do I know when to stop taking an extract?
Herbs work in a very individual way with the body. Some herbs act very quickly, while others take more time to balance, nourish and support body systems. Certain herbs are best taken for a short time (one to three weeks) while other herbs will yield their best results when they are taken for longer periods (one to six months or more). When duration is specifically important, it will be noted in the dosage recommendations in the **Herbal Repertory** (Chapter 7).

The following types of considerations determine duration. In general, the stronger the herb, the shorter the length of time it should be taken. Examples of these strong herbs include Chaparral, Lomatium and Uva Ursi. Other herbs, such as Gingko, Hawthorn, Oat Seeds and St. John's Wort, must be taken for a least one month before they even begin to share their healing qualities with us: therefore, these herbs should not be pulsed. In fact, many of these herbs should be taken for months in order to achieve best results.

Formulas designed to be taken for acute diseases, such as Golden Seal/Echinacea Complex™ for colds and flu, should be taken for shorter amounts of time. On the other hand, formulas aimed at chronic problems, such as Deprezac™ for depression, require longer periods of ingestion, as their benefits accrue over time.

When you are treating a problem that has existed for a long time, it is sometimes helpful to alternate between two formulas. Using acne as an example, take Acnetonic™ for one month and then take Dermatonic™ for one month. Start again with the Acnetonic™ and keep cycling every other month until the problem is resolved.

If duration is not indicated, then take the herb until symptoms cease. If you are in doubt, consult a knowledgable herbalist, a naturopath or medical doctor. Keep in mind that herbs are medicine and recommended dosages should not be exceeded.

Q: Since I am dealing with several different health problems, what is the best way to take herbs for different problems at the same time?

When taking different herbs for different health problems, there are four points to keep in mind. These guidelines are applicable to all age groups.

1) Go to the root cause of your problems rather than just treating separate symptoms. For example, a person may experience difficulty sleeping, digestive troubles, mouth ulcers, constipation and nervousness. If you treat each symptom as a separate problem, you will need herbs for sleep, stomach, mouth and the intestinal system, as well as herbs for the nervous system. What may be needed instead are herbs targeted at stress. Or it may be that the best system to strengthen is the digestive system if that is where the root cause of the separate symptoms is centered. When the root cause is addressed with appropriate herbs, then the other symptoms will disappear.

2) Take herbs for different problems at different times. Take herbs for the same problem at the same time. For example, if you

Milk Thistle

want to take Arthrotonic™ for arthritis and Feverfew for migraine headaches, I suggest that you take them at least fifteen minutes apart. On the other hand, if you are taking different herbs for the same problem, such as Dandelion, Burdock and Nettle for skin problems, they can be combined and taken at the same time. See item 4 below regarding guidelines for how many extracts to take at once.

3) Take herbs at least fifteen minutes apart. See item 2 above.

4) It is best to address no more than three health problems at once. Let's say you are taking herbs for asthma, arthritis and migraines, but you also suffer from skin rashes and chronic fatigue. At any given time, you must decide which three conditions to address, and then you'll need to take your herbs for those conditions at least fifteen minutes apart. It is okay to take a single extract, like Feverfew, for your migraines, and also to take combinations, like Adrenotonic™ for your asthma, and Arthrotonic™ for your arthritis. Just take them apart from each other.

Q: Can I take herbal extracts at the same time I am taking conventional drugs?
Yes. In many instances taking herbs at the same time as conventional drugs will actually support and heal the body faster and more thoroughly. For example, taking immune stimulating herbs while a person is on antibiotics is recommended, because these herbs will strengthen the immune system and prevent relapses after the round of antibiotics is done.

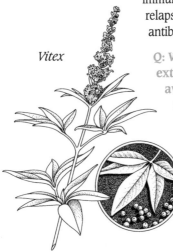

Vitex

Q: Why do some extracts taste so awful?
Don't let taste keep you from enjoying the healing benefits of herbs. In our society, we are addicted to two basic tastes: salty and sweet. But there are three

other tastes that are equally important in maintaining health: sour, bitter and pungent. These tastes, when taken as herbs or foods, initiate body reactions that help restore health. For example bitter herbs, such as Barberry root, help tone the stomach. Pungent tasting herbs, such as Turmeric, help tone the liver. It is possible to ingest herbs in capsule form to avoid the taste, but the digestive benefits the herbs offer are greatly minimized when they are in capsulized form. It is important to remember that herbs, even though they may not taste salty or sweet, put us in touch with Nature's pure energy to assist us in our quest for health.

Q: What is the best way to disguise the taste of liquid herbal extracts?

The best way to take extracts without affecting their healing properties is to put them in water, juice, and/or herbal tea, as long as the tea doesn't contain caffeine. Although some people prefer to put undiluted extracts directly in their mouths, putting extracts in some form of liquid is easier for most people. It is best to put herbs taken for digestion in two or three ounces of water.

Q: Can I give liquid herbal extracts to my children?

There are four things you must be aware of with children.

1) Children should be at least one year old before being given herbs. For children under a year old, you should give the extract only under the supervision of a knowledgeable herbalist or primary care physician (medical doctor, naturopath, acupuncturist, etc.). In a few instances in the **Herbal Repertory** (Chapter 7), reference is made to certain herbs which can be given to babies. These are Chamomile, Fennel, Pau D'Arco and Stomach Tonic™. See specific dosage instructions under these listings.

2) A child's dosage is a fraction of the adult dosage. If an extract calls for a 20 drop dose for an adult, adjust the dosage by giving two drops per year of age to a child. For example, a three-year-old child would take six drops of the extract (20 = 2 drops X 3 years old = 6 drops). If the extract calls for a 10 drop dose for an adult, adjust the dosage by giving one drop per year of age. Therefore, a three-year-old child would take three drops of the extract (10 = 1 drop X 3 years old = 3 drops). In the **Herbal**

Repertory (Chapter 7) California Poppy, Horsetail, Passion Flower and Red Clover are exceptions to this rule. See specific dosage instructions under these listings.

A second way to figure out a child's dosage is to divide the adult dosage by 150 pounds and multiply the answer by the *weight of the child*. For example, take an adult dosage of 30 drops and divide by 150 pounds = 2/10 of a drop, multiplied by the weight of a 30 pound child = 6 drops.

3) If the child is of slight build or is underweight for his/her age, determine the correct dosage by the weight of the child according to the formula above.

4) If the child has a weak constitution, i.e. is frail, recuperating from an illness or is in any weakened state, cut the usual child's dosage by 25-50 percent. Gauge dosage according to effectiveness.

Q: How can I get my child to take liquid herbal extracts?
Putting the drops in orange juice is the easiest way to give an herbal extract to a child, as orange juice best disguises the taste. Other juices may also do the trick.

Q: Can I give liquid herbal extracts to my pets? How much should I give them?
I have found over the years that pets respond very favorably to extracts. However, in the same way that you need to adjust dosages for children, care should be taken to adjust dosages for animals. The general rule is to give two drops per 10 pounds of weight. The best way to give extracts to pets is to mix it in their food. It is not necessary to evaporate the alcohol, as the amount of alcohol in a dose is too small to hurt them.

Q: How much alcohol will I get when I ingest an average dose of a liquid herbal extract?
A: Although some people may be concerned about the level of alcohol content in herbal extracts, there is little cause for worry. On average, 30 drops of an extract containing 70 percent alcohol (see the label on the bottle for percentage of alcohol) has the same amount of alcohol as one ripe banana. In addition, when you eat fruit, your body naturally produces alcohol via the fermentation process in your stomach. The main point I am emphasiz-

ing here is that the total amount of alcohol ingested from a 30 drop dose is very small.

Q: If I prefer to evaporate the alcohol out of an extract, how do I do that? Will evaporating the alcohol lessen the effectiveness of the extract in any way?

Evaporating the alcohol out of an herbal extract is best done on a dose-by-dose basis. Do not heat up an entire bottle of herbs as that can damage the herbs in the extract. Instead, add as many drops of the extract as are recommended per dosage to a cup of boiling water, or, if you wish, to an herbal tea that is naturally caffeine-free. Let the mixture sit for 5-10 minutes. Forty to 60 percent of the alcohol will evaporate during that time. In an extract containing 70 percent alcohol, the remaining alcohol will be about the same amount as you would find in a third of a ripe banana. Evaporating the alcohol in this manner does not in any way diminish the effectiveness of the herbs.

Q: How many drops should I take?

As a rule of thumb, follow the dosages suggested in the **Herbal Repertory** (Chapter 7) under the appropriate herb. You may want to modify suggested dosages under two circumstances. In the acute stage of an illness (at the beginning of a cold, for example), you should take fewer drops of an extract more frequently (every hour or two, for two to five days). In a chronic stage (during a long standing disease, such as arthritis), take the full dosage two or three times a day for much longer periods of time (one to six months).

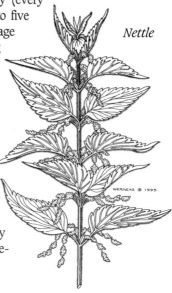

Nettle

Q: How many drops are in a one-ounce bottle of liquid herbal extract?

There are approximately 1,200 drops in a one-ounce bottle.

Q: How long will a one-ounce bottle of a liquid herbal extract last me?

It depends on the recommended daily dosage. Since there are approximately 1,200 drops in a one-ounce bottle of liquid herbal extract, you need to divide that number by the number of drops that you intend to take in one day in order to get the total number of days a one-ounce bottle will last you. For example, if you take 20 drops of Adrenotonic™ twice a day, your one-ounce bottle will last 30 days (1,200 drops total divided by 40 drops each day).

Q: How do I compare capsules to liquid herbal extracts? How do milligrams compare to drops?

It is difficult to compare capsules to extracts, especially when it comes to issues concerning assimilation and potency. With capsules, the body first has to break down plant fibers, and then digest and assimilate the plant constituents. If a person taking capsules has any digestive problems, breaking down and assimilating the herbs will be incomplete. In the case of liquid extracts, the body assimilates them more rapidly and thoroughly.

On the issue of potency, capsules lose potency through evaporation, oxidation and degradation, both in the manufacturing process and every day that they sit on the shelf. On the other hand, because they are processed immediately after harvesting and their active constituents are preserved in alcohol, extracts will keep their potency for a *minimum* of three years. Capsules cannot rival that.

The following equivalencies approximately translate capsule milligrams to liquid herbal extract drops:

25 mg = 1 drop

50 mg = 2 drops

500 mg = 20 drops

Approximately sixty 500 mg capsules = 1200 drops

(a one-ounce bottle)

Notes

Echinacea angustifolia

Chapter 5:
Deciding When to Avoid Certain Herbs

Q: What are "contraindications"?

The word "contraindication" is defined by *Tabor's Cyclopedic Medical Dictionary* (1977) as "any symptom or circumstance indicating the inappropriateness of a form of treatment otherwise advisable." Considering the hundreds of medicinal herbs available, not many have contraindications. *When a contraindication is noted in the **Herbal Repertory** (Chapter 7), it means you must alter your dosage as recommended, or you should not take that herb if you have the condition that is contraindicated. Pay strict attention to the directions given with each herb.*

By far, the most common contraindication relevant to the use of herbs is when pregnancy is involved, because some herbs have a direct influence on the uterus. Two of the ways herbs may affect a pregnancy in progress is by restricting the amount of blood reaching the uterus, or by stimulating uterine contractions. Other herbs are contraindicated while the baby is breast-feeding because some of the herbs' constituents may migrate into and through the milk to the infant. In terms of other health conditions, some herbs are contraindicated during acute inflammation because they can actually cause more damage than good at that stage. For example, Juniper Berries are contraindicated during acute urinary tract infection, as they can increase the inflammation that is already present.

Q: What is a "side effect"? Do herbs have side effects like drugs?

Tabor's Cyclopedic Medical Dictionary defines a "side effect" as "the action or effect, usually of a drug, other than that desired." Very few herbs have drug-like side effects. This is one of the primary reasons that so many people are turning to herbs as their preferred mode of treatment.

However, there are a few herbs listed in this book that may cause side effects, if taken in larger amounts than recommended. In addition, there is always the possibility that in a few cases, some people may have unpredictable reactions to herbs. Pay close attention to the dosage directions and all applicable notations regarding contraindications and side effects in the **Herbal Repertory** (Chapter 7). The following list summarizes possible side effects of herbs listed in this book:

Herb – Side Effect

Arnica – skin rash

Bionic Tonic™ – insomnia

Black Cohosh – mild frontal headache

Blue Cohosh – mid-cycle spotting & cramping

Cayenne – stomach and intestinal irritation

Chlorophyll Concentrate™ – dark green stools

Congest Free™ – insomnia, nervousness, loss of appetite, nausea, tremor, high blood pressure

Cran-Bladder ReLeaf™ – peculiar urine smell and color

Decongestonic™ – insomnia, nervousness, loss of appetite, nausea, tremor, high blood pressure

Chinese Kirin Red Ginseng – insomnia

Ephedra (Ma Huang) – insomnia, nervousness, loss of appetite, nausea, tremor, high blood pressure

HB Pressure Tonic™ – low blood pressure

Hops – depression (with long term usage)

Juniper Berries – may aggravate inflammation

Kidney Tonic™ – peculiar urine smell and color

Licorice – high blood pressure

Lobelia – nausea, vomiting, slowed respiration and heartbeat

Lomatium – skin rash

Pleurisy Root – nausea, vomiting

Uva Ursi – stomach irritation

Valerian – depression (with long term usage)

Golden Seal

WERNEKE © 1993

Q: If I am pregnant or breast-feeding, what precautions should I use when taking herbs?

Here is a list of herbs and herbal formulas that should be avoided during pregnancy and breast-feeding unless specifically recommended by a knowledgeable herbalist, naturopath or other primary care physician. Be sure to note the recommendations and contraindications listed with each herb in the **Herbal Repertory** (Chapter 7).

Herbs to avoid in pregnancy

Single extracts and formulas are listed separately

Single herbs not to be taken during pregnancy

Barberry

Black Cohosh (Not in the first seven months.)

Black Walnut Hulls

Blueberry

Blue Cohosh (Not in the first seven months.)

Catnip

Chaparral

Dong Quai

Ephedra (Ma Huang)

Golden Seal

Gravel Root

Juniper Berries

Licorice

Lobelia

Motherwort

Myrrh

Osha

Pennyroyal

Pleurisy Root

Shepherd's Purse

Turmeric

Uva Ursi

Vitex

Yarrow

Skullcap

WERNEKE © 1993

Formulas not to be taken during pregnancy

Acnetonic™

Adrenotonic™

Arthrotonic™
Bionic Tonic™
Cardiotonic™
Cholesterotonic™
Congest Free™
Cran-Bladder ReLeaf™
Cycle 1 Estrotonic™
Cycle 2 Progestonic™
Decongestonic™
Dermatonic™
Digestonic™
Essiac Tonic™
Golden Seal/Echinacea Complex™
HB Pressure Tonic™
Herbaprofen™
Kidalin™, Child and Adult Formulas
Kidney Tonic™
Liver Tonic™
Lymphatonic™
Menopautonic™
Montezuma's ReLeaf™
M-Roid ReLeaf™
Nervine Tonic™
Osha Root Complex Syrup™ (Not in the first three months.)
Para-Free™
PMS ReLeaf™
Respiratonic™
Smoke Free Drops™
Stomach Tonic™
Vein Tonic™
Yeast ReLeaf™

Herbs to avoid while breast-feeding
Single extracts and formulas listed together

Black Cohosh
Congest Free™
Decongestonic™
Ephedra (Ma Huang)
Gravel Root
Herbaprofen™
Para-Free™

Q: Besides during pregnancy and breast-feeding, are there precautions around taking herbs for people who have other pre-existing physical conditions?

Yes, there are two points to keep in mind. Is the person taking herbs also being treated with prescription or over-the-counter medication? Or is the person elderly, or very young?

1) If you are taking conventional medication for a health problem, be aware that taking herbs that work on the same problem may increase the effect of the drugs. For example, if you are taking medication to lower your blood pressure and you start taking herbs that do the same thing, you may find that your blood pressure decreases too much. Always monitor the results of taking any medications with your doctor and/or a person knowledgeable about herbs.

2) For children, especially those under the age of five, and also for adults over the age of 75, special care should be taken when administering herbs. Children and the elderly may be susceptible either to diarrhea or to overstimulation from certain herbs. Therefore it is important to start with smaller dosages and to monitor the reaction. You will find that in most instances everything will be normal. But in a few cases, diarrhea, skin rash, or other symptoms may occur, indicating the need to lessen dosages or to stop giving herbs altogether.

Q. Should I tell my doctor I am taking herbs?

Even though it might be difficult to talk to your doctor about the herbs that you may be taking, I think it is important to let him/her know what you are doing. While some doctors believe that herbs are dangerous or, conversely, have no effects, other doctors may already be knowledgable. Many M.D.s are now very curious about herbs, but they do not know where to find accurate, appropriate and useful information, in which case sharing this book may be helpful to both of you. Education is the key, and this book is a good beginning.

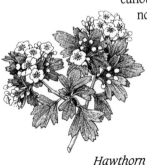

Hawthorn

Chapter 6:

Targeting Herbs for Specific Complaints

Q: What does "targeting" herbs mean?

"Targeting" means using the most therapeutically-focused herb at a specific time for a precise health problem. The herbal recommendations in this chapter were born out of my frustration that most sources of information on herbs do not differentiate clearly enough between various herbs usually suggested for a particular health problem. I view each herb as having a wide range of action; that is, an herb will affect the body at many different points during a disease. With the image of darts hitting a target in mind, I see each herb as a dart which gives you higher numbers of points the closer you get to using its main strengths at the right time in the course of a disease. Hitting the "bullseye" is when you derive the maximum benefit from an herb.

In relation to treating colds and flu, Golden Seal provides us with an example of how targeting is a tool that gives you stronger, faster and longer-lasting results. Presently, most Golden Seal is being consumed in herbal products that are used either for the prevention of colds and flu, or for the very beginning phases of colds and flu. Taking Golden Seal for these purposes is just hitting the outer ring of the target, because only 10 percent to 40 percent of Golden Seal's therapeutic benefits are being tapped as a preventative. The rest of Golden Seal's benefits are being wasted. Golden Seal hits the bullseye when you use it to combat inflammation that often starts on day three of a cold.

How to get the most out of this chapter:

Refer to the **Herbal Repertory** (Chapter 7) for a description of the healing actions, dosage recommendations, and contraindications and side effects, when applicable, for each recommended herb. *Pay special attention to the fact that several of the herbs recommended in these charts are contraindicated in pregnancy and some are contraindicated in breast-feeding.*

Herbs for Skin Problems

Skin problems can occur due to a multitude of factors including diet, stress, allergies, contact with irritating substances and even monthly hormonal changes. Many of the drugs used for skin problems tend to suppress symptoms so problems tend to recur. In order to rectify skin problems, you need to change how your body processes and eliminates waste products. In holistic herbal therapy, it is said that there is a one to ten ratio between the time it takes to heal a problem and how long a problem has existed. For example, if you have had psoriasis for twenty years, it may take up to two years for your skin to be problem-free. So, be aware that it may take a few weeks to many months to change your pattern but it is possible with persistence.

Symptoms	Recommended Herbs	
	Singles	*Formulas*
Dry flaky skin, eczema, psoriasis	**Pleurisy Root**	**Dermatonic**™
Oozy, wet skin, eczema, psoriasis	**Dandelion**	**Dermatonic**™
Acne, especially for teens eating fatty foods and sugar	**Burdock**	**Acnetonic**™
Acne and herpes around lips, worse around menstruation	**Vitex**	**Cycle 2 Progestonic**™
Fungus, lichen, Athlete's foot, candida	**Black Walnut**	**Yeast ReLeaf**™
Herpes, labial or genital	**Myrhh**	**Mouth Tonic**™
Shingles, rash in	**Red Clover**	**Dermatonic**™
Shingles, pain in	**Skullcap**	**Dermatonic**™
Diaper rash	**Pau D'Arco**	**Yeast ReLeaf**™
Poison Ivy, Poison Oak, Contact Dermatitis	**Red Root**	Internally: **Lymphatonic**™ Externally: **Ivy Itch ReLeaf**™
Hives, allergies; stop skin inflammation	**Nettle**	**Allertonic**™

Herbs for Poor Sleep

Match your "type" of insomnia or poor sleep patterns listed on the left under Symptoms to the recommended herbal extracts on the right. Strength classifications from "1" to "4" are also indicated for the herbs. A "4" classification is as strong as an herbal product can be (short of prescription medicine). Unlike Over the Counter (OTC) sleeping aids, these herbs do not suppress the dream state (also known as rapid eye-movement [REM] sleep).

Symptoms	Recommended Herbs (1=low to 4=high)	
	Singles	*Formulas*
Insomnia from being high strung; difficult time falling asleep	**Chamomile** (1)	
Sleep problems from muscle twitches & hyper-sensitive states	**Skullcap (1.75)**	
Insomnia from excessive mental stimulation	**Passion Flower** (2)	
Sleep disturbance with heart palpitation, digestive problems & headaches	**Valerian** (3)	
Long standing sleep disturbances; major difficulty falling asleep or staying asleep	**California Poppy** (4)	
Multiple sleep disturbance symptoms		**Deep Sleep™** (4) (Combines Chamomile, Passion Flower, Valerian, California Poppy & three other herbs)

Herbs for Colds and Flu

In this table, the symptoms associated with colds and flu are listed in chronological order in terms of what happens to the body in a typical cold cycle. To prevent yourself from getting a cold in the first place, it is important to use the herbs recommended for prevention. But if you are already feeling the symptoms of a cold, this table will help you choose which herbs you need to take for your specific symptoms, at the point you are in the cold cycle. For instance, Golden Seal is great for combatting inflammation on the second or third day of a cold. It does not work effectively to prevent colds, as Astragalus does, or cleanse the body after a cold, as Red Root does. Effective herbal treatment of colds and flu depends on when you take what herbs.

Cycle/Symptoms	Recommended Herbs	
	Singles	*Formulas*
Prevention; ongoing, way in advance of cold season		**Deep Chi Builder**™
Prevention; one to two months before cold season and/or during stressful periods	**Astragalus**	**Echinacea/ Astragalus Complex**™
Day one of cold/flu; whole body feeling achy, feverish	**Echinacea**	**Triple Source Echinacea**™
Day two or three; whole body feeling rotten; beginning of sore throat & inflammation	**Golden Seal**	**Golden Seal/ Echinacea Complex**™
Day four, five or six; cold/flu begins to infect particular area of body, i.e. mucus in the lungs	**Osha**	**Respiratonic**™
Day four, five or six; cold/flu begins to infect particular area of body, i.e. throat; coughing	**Wild Cherry**	**Osha Root Complex Syrup**™
Day four, five or six; sore throat with laryngitis & pharyngitis	**Collinsonia**	**Singer's Saving Grace**™
Day four, five or six; cold settles in the head; runny nose, thin mucus	**Ephedra & Mullein**	**Decongestonic**™
Day four, five or six; cold settles in head; dry membranes, thick mucus	**Ephedra & Yerba Mansa**	**Congest Free**™
The really hard-to-shake or recurring cold/flu	**Red Root**	**Lymphatonic**™

Herbs for Stopping Smoking

The first thing to consider in the process of stopping smoking is your motivation. I have seen over and over that no amount of herbs will make up for weak motivation, which often occurs when smokers are trying to quit in order to please others. If you truly want to quit for yourself out of choice, not obligation, then your likelihood of success dramatically increases. Because nicotine addiction affects the physiology of the body in several ways, it is best to provide yourself with herbal support in a variety of areas. This table lists symptoms in six basic areas—cravings, lung congestion, nervous irritablility, the weakened endocrine system, the digestive process and blood sugar balance. None of these herbs are habit forming.

Symptoms	Recommended Herbs	
	Singles	*Formulas*
Cravings; addictive alkaloids stored all over the body	Lobelia	
Lung congestion; choking feeling due to lung mucus	Osha	
Lung congestion	Pleurisy Root	
Nervous irritability; feeling as if you want to crawl out of your skin	Oat Seeds	
Nervous irritability; "chattering," busy brain	Passion Flower	
Weakened endocrine system contributes to cravings & low energy	Licorice	
Overall herbal formula for across-the-board body support		Smoke Free Drops™ (Combines Lobelia, Oat Seeds, Licorice, Osha, Pleurisy Root & three other herbs)
Poor digestion; constipation	Gentian	Digestonic™
Blood sugar imbalance; symptoms of hypoglycemia in initial stages of stopping smoking	Woodsgrown American Ginseng	

Herbs for Allergies

Because allergies, or allergic rhinitis, can be related to a multitude of seasonal and non-seasonal irritants ranging from tree pollens to house dust, this is a difficult area to address from just one vantage point. Generally, in addition to herbal support, I urge you to take corrective measures to reduce stress in your life (sinuses and nasal membranes react to overall health and stress levels) and to improve your overall diet (dairy products and grains, especially wheat, sugar, alcohol and sweets aggravate allergies), among other things. This table addresses the symptoms that most allergy sufferers can relate to, as well as designates what herbs are good for prevention and adrenal support, in the case of high stress. For those who wish to go into more detail, I recommend the following book: *Breathe Free* by Daniel Gagnon and Amadea Morningstar, published in 1990 by Lotus Press, Santa Fe, New Mexico.

Symptoms	Recommended Herbs	
	Singles	*Formulas*
Prevention of hay fever sensitivity to trees, flowers & ragweeds; also during hay fever season	**Nettle**	Allertonic™
Prevention & support; adrenal glands working overtime	**Siberian Ginseng**	Adrenotonic™
Liver support to help process inflammation that is clogging the body	**Barberry**	Liver Tonic™
Hay fever symptoms; sinus pain; thin mucus; lots of fluids!	**Ephedra & Mullein**	Decongestonic™
Hay fever symptoms; thick mucus; congestion; nothing is moving!	**Ephedra & Yerba Mansa**	Congest Free™
Asthma related to sensitivity to pollens	**Ephedra**	Congest Free™

Herbs for Digestive Problems

As stated in my discussion of the Ten Elements of Good Health (Chapter 1), it is extremely important for you to attend to the quality of your diet on a daily basis; however, if you are experiencing digestive problems, there are many herbs that are very effective aids to digestive system functions. Remember to practice good dietary habits and support your herbal treatments by drinking a lot of water (64 ounces a day).

Symptoms	Recommended Herbs	
	Singles	*Formulas*
Dry mouth; coated teeth & tongue in the morning	**Cayenne**	**Digestonic™**
Lack of stomach digestive enzymes, creating poor digestion; bloating after eating; indigestion	**Gentian**	**Digestonic™**
Stomach gas; bloating & burning sensation	**Chamomile**	**Stomach Tonic™**
Stomach or intestinal cramping with possible diarrhea	**Cramp Bark**	**Cramp ReLeaf™**
Poor fat absorption; oily stools; dry skin due to lack of liver bile secretion	**Barberry**	**Liver Tonic™**
Diarrhea	**Bayberry**	**Montezuma's ReLeaf™**
Candida symptoms; dermatitis; diarrhea, flatulence &"sick all over" feeling	**Pau D'Arco**	**Yeast ReLeaf™**
Sea sickness; motion sickness; nausea (even from chemotherapy or vertigo)	**Ginger**	

Passion Flower

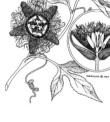

Herbs for Women's Reproductive System Problems

Among the various populations of people seeking alternative therapies, women are emerging as a major force in support of herbal medicine, specifically due to their need to find safer, less intrusive and less disruptive treatments for female reproductive system issues. Herbs answer this need because they offer a more harmonious and gentler way of working with the body. This table groups recommended herbs into four categories—herbs for menstrual distress, cycle balancing, menopause and sexual encounter infections.

Symptoms	Recommended Herbs	
	Singles	*Formulas*
Menstrual cramps, sharp	Cramp Bark	Cramp ReLeaf™
Menstrual cramps, dull; pain down the leg	Black Cohosh &/or Blue Cohosh	
Menstrual cramps, sharp; pain in muscles	Meadowsweet	Herbaprofen™
Delayed menstruation due to travel, cold, stress	Pennyroyal	
PMS symptoms; water retention; mood swings	Vitex & Dandelion	PMS ReLeaf™ or Cycle 2 Progestonic™
Cycle imbalance; lack of menstruation after getting off the pill	Dong Quai & Vitex	Alternate Cycle 1 Estrotonic™ & Cycle 2 Progestonic™
Cycle imbalance; breast, ovarian, uterine cysts	Red Root	Lymphatonic™
Cycle imbalance; estrogen enhancer; day 1 of menses to day 14	Black Cohosh or Dong Quai	Cycle 1 Estrotonic™
Cycle imbalance; progesterone enhancer day 15 of cycle to day 28	Vitex	Cycle 2 Progestonic™
Menopausal symptoms	Black Cohosh, Dong Quai or Vitex	Menopautonic™
Urinary tract infection after sex	Uva Ursi	Cran-Bladder ReLeaf™
Discomfort from herpes outbreak; lesions	Echinacea	Passion Potion™

Chapter 7:
Herbal Repertory

Notes on this Herbal Repertory:

This section lists single extracts and formulas in alphabetical order. To find the herbs that are best suited to your health issues, you can read the description of each herb in this section. Or better yet, you can start with the **Health Condition Index**, which recommends the best herbal extracts for conditions ranging from Abdominal Pain to Yeast Infection, and then refer back to this section to look up the specific herbs you need.

Note that when an herb is designated as a "fresh herb," it means the herb has not been dried. Also, for all formulas, ingredients are listed in descending order of content.

Please heed all dosage recommendations, including when and how to pulse dosages, and note contraindications and/or side effects, when applicable.

Notes on Pulsing

"Pulsing" is when you take an herb for a certain length of time and then stop for a while, in order to allow your body to work on its own without intervention during the rest period. Two-thirds of herbs should be pulsed to receive the maximum benefits. One-third are best not pulsed.

There are two possible ways of pulsing. For herbs you are taking for *short* or *long* periods of time, take for five days, stop for two days, and then repeat. For herbs you are taking for *long* periods of time, take for three weeks, stop for one week, and then repeat. Please note that some of the dosages indicated in this **Herbal Repertory** recommend specific pulsing periods.

If pulsing is not recommended for an herb, then that herb can be, or may *need* to be, taken continually for long periods of time to achieve results. See page 28 for a more complete explanation of pulsing.

Acnetonic™ (Burdock/Violet Complex). Specific for acne that occurs in adolescence or young adulthood. Also helpful for women who experience flare-ups of acne during hormonal shifts of their menstrual cycle or during ingestion of oral contraceptives.

Dose: *Take 20 drops three times a day for one month. Then take Dermatonic™ at the same dosage for the following month. Continue alternating Dermatonic™ and Acnetonic™ every other month. Best to pulse (see pages 28 & 49).*

Contraindications: *Not in pregnancy.*

Ingredients: *Burdock, Echinacea, Dong Quai, Sarsaparilla, Violet leaves, Oregon Grape root, Licorice, Dandelion root, Yellow Dock, Red Clover, Woodsgrown American Ginseng, Kelp.*

Adrenotonic™ (Black Currant/Licorice Complex). Superb adrenal gland tonic. Ideal formula to take after cortico-steroidal therapy. For any illnesses that are aggravated during stressful periods, such as asthma, Chronic Fatigue Immuno-Deficiency syndrome (CFIDS), hypoglycemia or allergies of all kinds. Prevents excessive response to everyday stress. A great female adaptogen as it will not disturb the menstrual cycle.

Dose: *Take 15-30 drops twice a day. Take for at least 100 days to achieve best results.*

Contraindications: *Not in pregnancy.*

Ingredients: *Black Currant leaves, Astragalus, Licorice, Siberian Ginseng, Woodsgrown American Ginseng, Schisandra, Sarsaparilla, Fo-ti.*

Alfalfa (*Medicago sativa*, fresh herb). High in chlorophyll. Excellent support for arthritis, rheumatism, colitis, ulcers,and anemia. A supportive herb to drink when taking sulfa or antibiotic drugs or when fasting.

Dose: *Take 15-30 drops up to four times a day.*

Allertonic™ (Nettle/Eyebright Complex). A formula used in cases of allergies that manifest as eczema, hay fever, hives, asthma, skin rash, sinusitis, headaches, allergic rhinitis, chronic bronchitis, itchy eyes, sneezing, inflammation of the mouth, stomach and/or intestines, diarrhea and, in some cases, arthritis. Prevents the release of inflammatory substances and reduces excessive body defense reactions.

Dose: *Take 20-40 drops two to three times a day. This*

formula is slow acting for some individuals. Take for a minimum of two weeks. If results are positive, continue for three to six months.

Ingredients: *Nettle, Licorice, Eyebright, Horehound, Osha, Horsetail, Mullein, Elecampane, Plantain.*

Arnica (*Arnica spp.*, fresh herbs). FOR EXTERNAL USE ONLY. A first aid liniment for muscular soreness and pain from sprains, bruises, strains, over-exertion; rheumatic pain, phlebitis or arthritis. Excellent for the sore "weekend warrior."

Use: *Apply every few hours; wash hands after applying.*

Contraindications: Do not apply on broken skin.

Side effects: Skin rash may develop. If the skin gets irritated, cease use.

Arthrotonic™ (Devil's Claw/Yucca Complex). Useful in reducing pain, inflammation, swelling, and tenderness of joints and muscles. Offers relief in arthritis, rheumatoid arthritis, myositis, fibromyalgia, irritable bowel syndrome, gout, or joint inflammation of synovial membranes (those covering the joints) and joint stiffness. Increases excretion and neutralization of uric acid and other waste products that initiate and prolong inflammation.

Dose: *Take 25 drops three times a day. Recommend pulsing (see pages 28 & 49) for three weeks on and stop for one week. Repeat cycle.*

Contraindications: *Not in pregnancy.*

Ingredients: *Devil's Claw, Burdock, Alfalfa, Black Cohosh, Licorice, Yucca, Echinacea, Pipsissewa, Wild Indigo, Horsetail.*

Black Cohosh

Astragalus (*Astragalus membranaceus [Huang Qi]*, dried root slice). Definitely one of the best preventative herbs available. Deep immune system tonic. Improves adrenal gland function.

WERNEKE © 1993

Useful for fatigue, frequent colds, or chronic non-healing sores. Increases production of interferon and increases resistance to viral infections.

Dose: *Take 15-30 drops twice a day. Take for 100 days or more to achieve best results.*

Barberry (*Berberis vulgaris,* dried root). As a bitter tonic, helps resolve indigestion and poor appetite. It improves nutrition by stimulating digestion, absorption and assimilation. Helpful for acne, psoriasis, herpes eruption and eczema, when these conditions are accompanied by constipation. Improves liver function. Also very useful in parasitic infection, especially giardia.

Dose: *As a bitter tonic, take 5 drops ten minutes before each meal. For other uses, take 10-20 drops three times a day. Best to pulse (see pages 28 & 49).*

Contraindications: *Not in pregnancy.*

Bayberry (*Myrica cerifera*, dried root bark). For long term inflammation of mouth, for bleeding gums, sore throat and stomach. For diarrhea from stress, excess food; for colitis or dysentery.

Dose: *Take 15-25 drops three times a day. For bleeding gums or sore throat, dilute, then gargle and swallow. Best to pulse (see pages 28 & 49).*

Bionic Tonic™ (Red Ginseng/Fo-ti Complex). Helps you stay awake, alert and mentally clear. Useful when driving, studying, doing a task over and over, or when you need to be alert, bushy-tailed and fully alive. Great as a mid-morning or mid-afternoon pick-me-up. Contains no caffeine or Ephedra (Ma Huang).

Dose: *Take 15-30 drops mid-morning, mid-afternoon, or other times as a pick-me-up. Best to pulse (see pages 28 & 49).*

Contraindications: *Not in pregnancy.*

Side effects: *Taking too close to bedtime may cause insomnia.*

Ingredients: *Chinese Kirin Red Ginseng, Fo-ti, Gotu Kola, Siberian Ginseng, Damiana, Woods-grown American Ginseng, Licorice, Prickly Ash berry, Peppermint, Ginger, Cayenne.*

Eyebright

Bitter Tonic™ (see Digestonic)

Black Cohosh *(Cimicifuga racemosa,* dried root*)*. For dull aching pains without acute inflammation in joints, muscles or uterus. For weak, irregular uterine contractions during labor or for after-birth pains. Useful for menopausal women experiencing hot flashes and depression.
Dose: *Take 10-20 drops every four hours. Best to pulse (see pages 28 & 49).*
Contraindications: *Not during the first seven months of pregnancy. Do not use while nursing.*
Side effects: *Excessive use may cause a mild frontal headache.*

Black Walnut/Wormwood Complex
(see Para-Free™)

Black Walnut Hull *(Juglans nigra,* fresh "green" hull*)*. For eczema, acne, lichen, candida, intestinal distress, diarrhea, chronic scaly skin diseases and inflammation of the mouth, throat and stomach.
Dose: *Take 10-20 drops up to three times a day. Not for long term use. Best to pulse (see pages 28 & 49). Externally: As a wash, one teaspoon of the extract in half a cup of boiled water. Apply when water cools.*

Blueberry *(Vaccinium myrtillus,* fresh leaf*)*. Useful for adult onset diabetes, the type that can be controlled by diet. Lowers elevated blood sugar level. Increases uric acid elimination and relieves gout. Stops diarrhea, especially in children.
Dose: *Take 20-30 drops after meals. Best to pulse (see pages 28 & 49).*
Contraindications: *Not in pregnancy.*
Note: *Not useful for insulin-dependent diabetics.*

Blue Cohosh *(Caulophyllum thalictroides,* dried root*)*. Use for menstrual cramps when dull pains extend to buttocks and back of legs. Facilitates childbirth when delay in labor is due to weakness, fatigue or lack of uterine power.
Dose: *Take 5-15 drops up to four times a day. Best to pulse (see pages 28 & 49).*
Contraindications: *Not during the first seven months of pregnancy.*
Side effects: *May cause mid-cycle spotting and cramping in sensitive women.*

Burdock (*Arctium lappa*, Autumn-gathered dried root). Effective in dry and scaly eczema, psoriasis, acne, dandruff and boils. Stimulates digestive juices and bile secretion. In gout, stimulates excretion of urea and uric acid.

Dose: *Take 15-25 drops three times a day for an extended period of time (three to four months).*

Burdock/Violet Complex (see Acnetonic™)

Butcher's Broom/Collinsonia Complex (see M-Roid ReLeaf™)

Calendula (*Calendula officinalis*, fresh flower). Internally: For peptic ulcers and inflammation of the mouth. Externally: For healing skin burns or inflammation, abrasions, pressure ulcers (i.e., bed sores), and impetigo.

Dose: *Take 10-15 drops up to four times a day. Best to pulse (see pages 28 & 49). Externally: Dilute with water and apply.*

California Poppy (*Eschscholzia californica*, fresh flowering plant). Specific for people who have difficulty falling asleep or who wake up during the night or too early in the morning. Permits deep sound sleep. Great for sleepless, frenetic children, or for children who sleep so soundly that they wet the bed.

Dose: *Take 20-40 drops one hour before sleep and again just before bedtime. For bed wetting, in children over five years old, use with Horsetail, 10 drops of each twice a day. Best to pulse (see pages 28 & 49).*

California Poppy/Valerian Complex (see Deep Sleep™)

Cardiotonic™ (Hawthorn/Motherwort Complex). Formula for heart irregularities with rapid heart beat episodes or weakness of heart muscle. Specific support for angina, as it greatly improves the blood flow to the heart muscle. Offers excellent support in almost all heart disease.

Note: *Not useful for damaged heart where the damage is termed organic. Works best for functional heart problems (i.e., angina).*

Dose: *Take 15-25 drops three times a day for one month, then twice a day for an unlimited period of time.*

Contraindications: *Not in pregnancy.*

Ingredients: *Hawthorn flowers, leaves and berries, Motherwort, Bugleweed, Ginkgo, Passion Flower, Woods-grown American Ginseng, Siberian Ginseng, Rosemary.*

Catnip (*Nepeta cataria*, fresh pre-flowering herb). Taken hot, stimulates sweating in colds and flu, and breaks up fevers. Taken cold, eases stomach and intestinal cramps in adults and especially in children. Eases insomnia caused by muscle tension.
Dose: *Take 20-30 drops up to five times a day. Best to pulse (see pages 28 & 49).*
Contraindications: *Not in pregnancy.*

Cat's Claw (*Uncaria tomentosa [Uña de Gato]*, dried tree bark). Europeans report positive clinical use with AZT in treating AIDS. Genital herpes and herpes zoster both respond favorably to its use. Also helpful for diverticulitis, hemorrhoids, colitis, leaky bowel syndrome, fistulas, peptic ulcers, gastritis, gastric ulcers, candidiasis, and Khron's disease. Cat's Claw helps to curb parasites and dysentery. Found useful in arthritis, bursitis, and rheumatism.
Dose: *Take 20-40 drops three to five times a day. Best to pulse (see pages 28 & 49).*

Cayenne (*Capsicum annuum*, dried fruit). In viral infections, cools dry, hot mucous membranes. Small amounts increase secretions; useful in case of dry mouth and a lack of digestive secretions due to nervousness, alcohol abuse, prescription drugs and old age. Stimulates circulation.
Dose: *Take 5-10 drops in warm water. Best to pulse (see pages 28 & 49).*
Side effects: *Large doses may irritate the stomach and intestines in sensitive people.*

Chamomile (*Matricaria recutita*, whole fresh flower). Internally: Useful for anxiety, insomnia, indigestion, flatulence, gastritis, stomach ulcers, gingivitis, gastro-enteritis, colitis and menstrual related migraines. Externally: Reduces inflammation and speeds up healing of wounds.
Dose: *For adults, take 20-50 drops up to four times a day. For babies, give 1-2 drops, diluted in a liquid, up to three times a day.*
Note: *Safe for babies two months and older.*

Chamomile/Catnip Complex (see Stomach Tonic™)

Chaparral (*Larrea tridentata*, dried leaf, flower and seed). Helpful in autoimmune and allergic disorders. For people who have been in long-term contact with chemicals, metals or aromatic hydrocarbons, such as solvents, paints and thinners. Also for poor digestion and assimilation of dietary fats.

Dose: *Take 20 drops up to three times a day. Best to pulse (see pages 28 & 49).*

Contraindications: *Not in pregnancy. Should not be used in large amounts by persons with pre-existing liver conditions such as hepatitis and cirrhosis. Discontinue use if nausea, fever, fatigue or jaundice (e.g. dark or yellow discoloration of the eyes) should occur.*

Chaste Tree Berries (see Vitex)

Chickweed (*Stellaria media*, fresh herb). Internally: Useful as a diuretic for PMS water retention and for overly acidic urine from excessive meat eating or steroid intake. Externally: Use as a rub for arthritis, rheumatism, sprains or gout.

Dose: *Take 15-25 drops three times a day. Externally: Dilute with water and apply.*

Chinese Kirin Red Ginseng (see Ginseng, Chinese Kirin Red)

Chlorophyll Concentrate™ (extracted from English Nettle). Use for low red blood cell count, fatigue, shortness of breath, high altitude sickness, or heavy menstrual flow. Intestinal deodorizer.

Dose: *Each 36 drop dose delivers 100 milligrams of Chlorophyll. Take 20-35 drops (before meals) three times a day.*

Side effects: *Dark green stools.*

Cholesterotonic™ (Siberian Ginseng/Devil's Claw Complex). For elevated cholesterol and/or triglyceride levels, especially during periods of physical or emotional stress. Helps to increase High Density Lipoproteins (HDL, the good cholesterol) and decrease Low Density Lipoproteins (LDL, the bad cholesterol). Also helpful when these elevations are due to excessive alcohol and/or fat intake.

Dose: *Take 20 drops three times a day after meals.*

Contraindications: *Not in pregnancy.*

Ingredients: *Siberian Ginseng, Devil's Claw, Woodsgrown American Ginseng, Greater Celandine, Fo-ti, Shepherd's Purse, Couchgrass, Virginia Snakeroot, Prickly Ash.*

Collinsonia (*Collinsonia canadensis*, Autumn-gathered fresh root). Useful for throat irritation from intensive talking, singing or shouting, as in pharyngitis and laryngitis. Also, for hemorrhoids and varicosities due to poor venous blood circulation with a sense of constriction, rectal pain and bladder irritation with painful urination.

Dose: Take 30-40 drops up to four times a day. For irritation of throat, dilute, then gargle and swallow. Best to pulse (see pages 28 & 49).

Collinsonia/Jack-in-the-Pulpit Complex (see Singer's Saving Grace™)

Congest Free™ (Ephedra [Ma Huang]/Yerba Mansa Complex). For sinus congestion with hot dry membranes, headache, pain, pressure and heaviness in the sinuses, low fever, blocked ears, earache and even bleeding nose from dryness. Take if mucus is thick, if it is difficult to blow your nose and if it feels like your head is in a vice-like grip. Good to use when you are congested and must travel by plane.

Dose: *For general usage, take 15-25 drops every four hours. Best to pulse (see pages 28 & 49). Do not take for more than six weeks in succession. If taken specifically for travel via plane, take 60-80 drops one hour prior to take off and also before landing.*

Contraindications: *Not in pregnancy or while nursing.*

Warning: *Because this formula contains Ephedra (Ma Huang), seek advice from a health care practitioner prior to use if you are pregnant or nursing; or if you have high blood pressure, heart or thyroid disease, diabetes, difficulty in urination due to prostate enlargement; or if taking an MAO inhibitor or any other prescription drug. NOT INTENDED FOR USE BY PERSONS UNDER 18 YEARS OF AGE. KEEP OUT OF THE REACH OF CHILDREN.*

Side effects: *May induce insomnia. Reduce or discontinue use if nervousness, tremor, sleeplessness, loss of appetite, nausea or high blood pressure occur.*

Ingredients: *Ephedra [Ma Huang], Yerba Mansa, Cubeb berries, Eyebright, Osha, Cayenne.*

WERNEKE © 1993

Feverfew

Cool Kava Complex™ (Kava Kava/Chamomile Complex). Useful for anxiety, edginess, tension, mental and physical agitation, as well as for other symptoms of nervousness and high level stress. Helps relax muscle tension due to stress. Permits sleep when insomnia is due to muscle and mental tension. Acts as a mood elevator; is useful in depression where there is a lot of agitation, anxiety and inability to relax.
Dose: *Take 25 drops two to four times a day. Chronic situations may require long term use. If taken for depression, consider alternating with Deprezac™.*
Ingredients: *Kava Kava, Chamomile, St. John's Wort, Oat seeds, Passion Flower, Hops, Skullcap, Stevia.*

Cramp Ban™ (see Cramp ReLeaf™)

Cramp Bark (*Viburnum opulus*, dried root bark). Calms painful menstruation with stabbing-like pains, severe discomfort and abundant bleeding. Calms the stomach, intestines, heart and nervous system. Useful for morning sickness and for threatened miscarriage in the last trimester.
Dose: *Take 20-60 drops up to every two hours if needed. Best to pulse (see pages 28 & 49).*

Cramp ReLeaf™ (Black Haw/Cramp Bark Complex). Relieves sharp, strong menstrual cramps occurring prior to or during menstruation. Calms diarrhea and upset stomach that accompany menstruation. Improves ovarian and uterine circulation, soothes the pelvic muscles and promotes toning of the entire birthing organ. Reduces morning sickness and controls after-birth pains. In combination with Shepherd's Purse, it prevents postpartum hemorrhage.
Dose: *Take 40-100 drops, or one-half to one teaspoon in warm water, every three or four hours. Best to pulse (see pages 28 & 49).*
Ingredients: *Black Haw, Cramp Bark, Beth Root, Cloves, Cinnamon, Wild Yam, Cardamom, Orange Peel.*

Cran-Bladder ReLeaf™ (Cranberry/Uva Ursi Complex). Prevents and stops recurring urinary tract infection (UTI), especially in females, in two ways: 1) prevents bacteria from sticking to the walls of the bladder, and 2) oils from the herbs help deactivate and destroy the bacteria that are present in the bladder, urethra, and urethers. Stimulates the immune system of the urinary tract, acidifies the urine and tones the urinary system. Specific for infection occurring after intercourse. Useful for frequent, urgent, burning or painful urination, lower back pain, pain in the pubic area, the tendency to urinate excessively at night, changes in the color of the urine, and decreases in the amount of the urine.

Dose: *For acute symptoms, take 20 drops every hour or two. For chronic conditions, take 30 drops twice a day for an unlimited amount of time as a preventative.*

Contraindications: *Not in pregnancy.*

Side effects: *Urine may have a peculiar smell and color.*

Ingredients: *Cranberry, Uva Ursi, Echinacea, Nettle, Buchu, Horsetail, Pipsissewa, Yarrow, Meadowsweet, Stevia.*

Cycle 1 Estrotonic™ Day 1-14 Support and Cycle 2 Progestonic™ Day 15-28 Support

These combinations were formulated to be used in tandem: for regulating menstrual cycles for women who are getting off oral contraceptives or who have erratic menstrual cycles due to a variety of interruptions such as breast feeding, physical reactions to travel, trauma, etc.; for women who are having difficulty conceiving; for women who have excessively long or short menstrual cycles. Three to six months of alternating Cycle 1 Estrotonic™ and Cycle 2 Progestonic™ will reestablish a normal, balanced cycle. These formulas work together over the course of the 28 day menstrual cycle and should be taken as follows.

Cycle 1 Estrotonic™ Day 1-14 Support (Black Cohosh/ Dong Quai Complex).

This formula specifically balances estrogen levels in order to reestablish proper timing of the menstrual cycle and to facilitate ovulation.

Dose: *Take 30 drops twice a day for the first half of the menstrual cycle. Begin taking from the first day of menstruation to the fourteenth day (ovulation). On the fifteenth day, switch to Cycle 2 Progestonic™.*

Contraindications: *Not in pregnancy.*

Ingredients: *Black Cohosh, Dong Quai, Shatavari, False Unicorn, Squaw Vine, Licorice, Woodsgrown American Ginseng, Stevia.*

Cycle 2 Progestonic™ Day 15-28 Support (Vitex/Wild Yam Complex).

This formula increases the production of progesterone in balance with estrogen levels established in the first half of the menstrual cycle. Aids conception, because increased progesterone promotes proper implantation of the fertilized egg. Can be taken specifically for PMS symptoms without alternating with Cycle 1 Estrotonic™; helps relieve water retention, swollen and tender breasts, lower backache, cramping, fatigue, irritability, insomnia, depression, difficulty in concentrating, panic attacks, anxiety, mood swings, crying, physical and emotional tension, low blood sugar, low sex drive, headaches and migraines.

Dose: Take 30 drops twice a day for the second half of the menstrual cycle. Begin taking on the fifteenth day of the menstrual cycle and continue until the first day of next menstruation. Then switch to Cycle 1 Estrotonic™. Keep alternating Cycle 1 Estrotonic™ and Cycle 2 Progestonic™ for three to six months to achieve best results. If used specifically for PMS symptoms rather than for regulation of menstrual cycle, begin taking 30 drops up to twice a day, 8-10 days prior to onset of menstruation.

Contraindications: *Not in pregnancy.*

Ingredients: *Vitex, Wild Yam, Dandelion, Reishi, Blue Cohosh, Chickweed, Shatavari, Black Haw, Cinnamon, Orange peel.*

Damiana (*Turnera spp.*, dried leaf). Has a reputation as an aphrodisiac. Useful in anxiety and depression. Use for irritation of urinary passages (urethra or bladder) from emotional stress, sexual stress, or stress due to traveling. For delayed menstruation in young girls.

Dose: *Take 20-40 drops in warm water three times a day. Best to pulse (see pages 28 & 49).*

Dandelion (*Taraxacum officinale*, fresh Autumn-gathered root, leaf and flower). For poor bile secretion, poor appetite and digestive function, constipation from lack of bile, rheumatic conditions, eczema, chronic skin eruptions, or psoriasis aggravated by emotional stress and/or

WERNEKE © 1993

Betony

fatty foods. As a potassium-rich diuretic, helpful for water retention due to heart problems, PMS or heat sickness.

Dose: *Take 20-40 drops three or four times a day.*

Dandelion/Uva Ursi Complex (see Kidney Tonic™)

Decongestonic™ (Ephedra [Ma Huang]/Mullein Complex). For head colds with runny nose, teary, itchy eyes, sneezing and postnasal drip. Use when there is a lot of thin moving clear mucus present. Excellent for hay fever, sinus inflammation, allergy-induced asthma or bronchitis. Dries out sinuses and respiratory passages.

Dose: *Take 15-30 drops every four hours. Best to pulse (see pages 28 & 49). Do not take for more than six weeks in succession.*

Contraindications: *Not in pregnancy or while nursing.*

Warning: *Because this formula contains Ephedra (Ma Huang), seek advice from a health care practitioner prior to use if you are pregnant or nursing; or if you have high blood pressure, heart or thyroid disease, diabetes, difficulty in urination due to prostate enlargement; or if taking an MAO inhibitor or any other prescription drug. NOT INTENDED FOR USE BY PERSONS UNDER 18 YEARS OF AGE. KEEP OUT OF THE REACH OF CHILDREN.*

Side effects: *May induce insomnia. Reduce or discontinue use if nervousness, tremor, sleeplessness, loss of appetite, nausea or high blood pressure occur.*

Ingredients: *Ephedra [Ma Huang], Mormon Tea, Mullein, Coltsfoot, Yerba Santa, Eyebright, Cubeb berries.*

Deep Chi Builder™ (Super Reishi/Shiitake Complex). High quality deep immune system toner. Has anti-cancer, anti-tumor, immunostimulating, and adaptogenic properties. Protects the liver, kidneys, stomach and heart. Useful in reducing high cholesterol and high triglycerides levels. Helps relieve nervousness, anxiety, sleeplessness, dizziness, chronic hepatitis, allergies, heart disease, high blood pressure, and stomach and intestinal ulcers, as well as chronic respiratory problems such as asthma, emphysema and bronchitis. Prevents blood clot formation and stabilizes blood sugar problems. Excellent support for HIV, ARC, and AIDS treatment, and as a cancer preventative or with orthodox cancer therapy. Helps to rebuild the body after long, serious or debilitating diseases. Helps prevent antibiotic-resistant bacterial infections.

Dose: *Take 20 to 30 drops twice a day for a minimum of* *one month. Best results are achieved by taking for 100 days or more, then stopping for one month before repeating.*

Ingredients: *Reishi & Shiitake mushrooms, California Spikenard, Astragalus, Maitake mushroom, Ashwagandha, Siberian Ginseng, Schisandra, Cordyceps, Ginger.*

Deep Sleep™ (California Poppy/Valerian Complex). Specific for inability to fall asleep, waking up during the night, or waking up too early in the morning. For insomnia resulting from depression, for waking up groggy or tired, as well as for fitful and/or agitated sleep. For sleep problems accompanied by cramps or pain. For insomnia while weaning from drugs, alcohol or cigarettes. Also for inability to fall asleep from tiredness. Helps to reeducate the brain sleep center.

Dose: *Take 30-60 drops one hour prior to sleep and again at bedtime. Works better the second or third night. Best to pulse (see pages 28 & 49).*

Ingredients: *California Poppy, Valerian, Passion Flower, Chamomile, Lemon Balm, Oat seeds, Orange peel.*

Deprezac™ (St. John's Wort/Lemon Balm Complex). Slow acting formula specific for mild to medium depression. Possesses sedative and anti-depressant effects. Decreases feelings of anxiety, tension, fatigue, irritability, depression, insomnia, agitation, loss of appetite, loss of interest and excessive sleeping. Useful for Seasonal Affective Disorder (SAD).

Dose: *Take 30 drops three times a day for three weeks, then 30 drops twice a day for at least six months.*

Contraindications: *Not effective for bi-polar syndrome and/or for any other severe pathologic depressive states. These conditions usually require conventional drugs.*

Ingredients: *St. John's Wort, Lemon Balm, Kola nuts, Oat seeds, Peppermint, Valerian, Siberian Ginseng, Rosemary, Damiana, Stevia.*

Dermatonic™ (Red Clover/Burdock Complex). Helpful for cases of eczema, psoriasis, contact dermatitis. Eases itching, oozing, thickening or scaling of the skin. Speeds up healing and development of smooth, pliable skin. Use with Allertonic™ if skin problem is due to allergic reaction. For acne, alternate with Acnetonic™.

Dose: *Take 20-30 drops three times a day. Best to pulse (see pages 28 & 49).*

Contraindications: *Not in pregnancy.*

Ingredients: *Red Clover, Burdock, Pleurisy Root, Dande-*

lion, Oregon Grape root, Echinacea, Gotu Kola, Butternut, Devil's Club, Blue Flag.

Devil's Claw (*Harpagophytum procumbens*, dried secondary tuber). Safe anti-inflammatory for arthritis, rheumatism, gout, joint inflammation, gall bladder problems with pancreatic distress, and for elevated cholesterol and uric acid blood levels.

Dose: *Take 30 drops three times a day. Recommend pulsing (see pages 28 & 49) for three weeks on and stop for one week. Repeat cycle.*

Devil's Claw/Yucca Complex (see Arthrotonic™)

Digestonic™ (Gentian/Angelica Complex). Slow but sure acting tonic for the stomach. Use for poor appetite, acid indigestion, and poor stomach or intestinal function. Specific for stomach ulcers, it reduces inflammation of the lining and normalizes secretions. Stimulates breakdown and assimilation of food nutrients. Use in anemia, nausea, vomiting or diarrhea, and recurring canker or mouth sores (aphtous stomatitis).

Dose: *Take 5-15 drops, ten to twenty minutes before meals. Best to pulse (see pages 28 & 49). Use Stomach Tonic™ between meals.*

Contraindications: *Not in pregnancy.*

Ingredients: *Gentian, Quassia, Angelica, Golden Seal, Bayberry, Cardamom.*

Dong Quai (*Angelica sinensis [Dang Qui]*, cured root slices). In deficient estrogen or testosterone secretion, it increases cellular uptake of these hormones in uterine, vaginal, ovarian or prostatic disorders. For menopausal distress. For PMS with dull aching pain before or during menstruation.

Dose: *Take 10-15 drops up to three times a day. Best to pulse (see pages 28 & 49).*

Contraindications: *Not in pregnancy. Not during acute inflammation of above-mentioned tissues.*

Dong Quai/Vitex Complex (see Menopautonic™)

Echinacea (*Echinacea angustifolia*, dried root). A must in the beginning stages of a cold or flu. Increases production, maturation and aggressiveness of white blood cells against intruders. Great on swollen areas due to bee, wasp, gnat and mosquito bites. Helps reduce swelling and stimulates repair of tendons, ligaments and muscle sheaths.

Excellent for tendonitis, bursitis, tennis elbow, skier's knee and jogger's ankle. Prevents or slows down bacterial and viral infections by strengthening connective tissues. Gets rid of dead microbes, dead cells and other waste products by stimulating lymphatic drainage.

Dose: *For acute symptoms, take 10-40 drops every hour. If chronic, take 20-40 drops up to four times a day. Best to pulse (see pages 28 & 49).*

Echinacea/Astragalus Complex™ A deep immune system activator. Best tonic to use during the change of seasons to support and boost the immune system. Helps prevent colds and flu by increasing interferon production (interferon alerts the body at the first sign of an infection and prepares the body to deal with invaders). Use to build the immune system before stressful times or while traveling. Helps prevent recurring middle ear infections (otitis media) in children. Also for acute tonsillitis, genital or oral herpes, upper respiratory tract infection. For chronic yeast infection, thrush and contact dermatitis.

Dose: *As a tonic, take 20 drops twice a day for 30 days. For acute symptoms, take 20 drops every hour. If chronic, take 15-20 drops three or four times a day. Best to pulse (see pages 28 & 49).*

Ingredients: *Fresh Echinacea angustifolia root and flowers, fresh Echinacea purpurea root, dried Echinacea angustifolia root, Astragalus, Osha, Calendula, dried Echinacea purpurea seed.*

Echinacea/Red Root Complex (see Lymphatonic™)

Echinacea, Triple Source (See Triple Source Echinacea™)

Elderberry (*Sambucus nigra*, fresh berry). Used traditionally as a spring cleanser. Helps get rid of excess mucous production. New research indicates it is helpful in deactivating the influenza virus. Taken in the early stages of flu, it prevents symptoms

Milk Thistle

W.BRNTKE © 1993

64

from taking hold.

Dose: *Take 40 drops every four hours at the first sign of the flu. Best to pulse (see pages 28 & 49).*

Ephedra (*Ephedra sinica [Ma Huang]*, dried twig). For hay fever, head colds, sinus congestion or allergy-induced asthma.

Dose: *Take 20 drops every four hours. Best to pulse (see pages 28 & 49). Do not take for more than six weeks.*

Contraindications: *Not in pregnancy or while nursing.*

Warning: *Because this formula contains Ephedra (Ma Huang), seek advice from a health care practitioner prior to use if you are pregnant or nursing; or if you have high blood pressure, heart or thyroid disease, diabetes, difficulty in urination due to prostate enlargement; or if taking an MAO inhibitor or any other prescription drug. NOT INTENDED FOR USE BY PERSONS UNDER 18 YEARS OF AGE. KEEP OUT OF THE REACH OF CHILDREN.*

Side effects: *May induce insomnia. Reduce or discontinue use if nervousness, tremor, sleeplessness, loss of appetite, nausea or high blood pressure occur.*

Note: *Ephedra (Ma Huang) should never be used as a stimulant, to "give" one energy, or for weight loss.*

Ephedra (Ma Huang)/Mullein Complex (see Decongestonic™)

Ephedra (Ma Huang)/Yerba Mansa Complex (see Congest Free™)

Essiac Tonic™ (Sheep Sorrel/Burdock Complex). This formula was originally given to Canadian nurse Rene Caisse by a Chippewa Indian. Helps move the body toward a state of integration and health. Alleviates and gets rid of chronic and degenerative diseases. Boosts the immune system, cleanses and supports the liver and the blood. Useful in autoimmune disorders, allergic disorders, and Chronic Fatigue Immuno-Deficiency Syndrome (CFIDS).

Dose: *If symptoms are acute, take 40 drops in two ounces of hot water twice a day, morning and evening, on an empty stomach for 32 days. Best to pulse (see pages 28 & 49) for 32 days on and one week off. Repeat cycle. For prevention, take for 32 days twice a year. Do not eat or drink anything for at least one hour after taking Essiac Tonic™.*

Contraindications: *Not in pregnancy.*

Ingredients: *Sheep Sorrel, Burdock, Slippery Elm, Turkey Rhubarb.*

Eyebright (*Euphrasia officinalis*, dried herb). Internally: Take for hay fever and allergies with watery eyes, sneezing, runny nose, frontal headache and stuffy sinuses. Externally: Use for rapid relief of redness and swelling in conjunctivitis or blepharitis.
Dose: *Internally: Take 20-30 drops every three hours. Best to pulse (see pages 28 & 49). Externally: Must dilute. Mix 20 drops in 1/4 cup hot water. Let water cool and use as a wash.*

Fennel (*Foeniculum vulgare*, dried seed). Eliminates flatulence. Very useful for babies who have gas and distressed digestive systems (i.e., diarrhea, dyspepsia, intestinal spasms). Increases milk secretion in nursing mothers.
Dose: *For adults, take 30-40 drops up to four times a day. For babies, give 1-2 drops, diluted in a liquid, up to three times a day.*
Note: *Safe for babies two months and older.*

Feverfew (*Tanacetum parthenium*, dried leaf). Use for neuralgia and for spasms of the alimentary canal (gut). Useful for migraine headaches, rheumatoid arthritis and psoriasis when taken for at least three months.
Dose: *Take 15-30 drops every day for migraine prevention or other symptoms. Can be taken for an unlimited period of time. Most acute migraine headaches may be stopped by taking 30 drops of the extract every half hour during attacks.*

Fo-ti (*Polygonum multiflorum [Ho shou wu]*, dried root slice). For physical debility, high cholesterol levels, and weakness. Long-term immune system tonic.
Dose: *Take 15-30 drops three times a day. Take for 100 days to achieve best results.*
Contraindications: *Not when diarrhea is present.*

Gentian (*Gentiana lutea*, dried root). For poor appetite, acid indigestion, poor stomach or intestinal function. Stimulates digestive function after prolonged illness. For anemia or when recuperating from nausea, vomiting or diarrhea.
Dose: *Take 5-15 drops in a little water at least 10 minutes before meals. Best to pulse (see pages 28 & 49).*
Contraindications: *Not when gastric and duodenal ulcers are present.*

Gentian/Angelica Complex (see Digestonic™)

Ginger (*Zingiber officinalis*, fresh root). Relieves motion sickness, nausea (even from chemotherapy or vertigo), vomiting and morning sickness better than "Dramamine™." Relieves indigestion, abdominal and menstrual cramping, dyspepsia and gastric hypoacidity. Helps with acute colds and flu.

Dose: *Take 10-20 drops three times a day before meals. Best to pulse (see pages 28 & 49). For motion sickness, take 30-60 drops thirty minutes before your trip. Repeat every two to four hours.*

Ginkgo (*Ginkgo biloba*, fresh Autumn-gathered yellowing leaf). Has a scavenging effect on free radicals. For hearing and sight disorders with poor blood flow in ears and eyes; tinnitus. Helpful for Alzheimer's disease, vertigo associated with inner ear problems; loss of memory and alertness. Helps prevent poor circulation problems in eyes, skin, and extremities when diabetes is present.

Dose: *Take 20-30 drops up to four times a day. Maximum benefits are achieved when used for at least six months to one year.*

Ginkgo/Gotu Kola Complex (see Remember Now™)

Ginseng, Chinese Kirin Red (*Panax ginseng*, cured dried root). Most stimulating of the Ginsengs. For physical or emotional stress or exhaustion, mild depression, tiredness. Very helpful to older people whose appetite, energy and stamina are low, especially while recuperating from disease or surgery.

Dose: *Take 5-20 drops two to three times a day. Best to pulse (see pages 28 & 49).*

Contraindications: *Not for use when thyroid disease, high blood pressure, hyperglycemia or insomnia are present.*

Side effects: *If taken too close to bedtime, may cause insomnia.*

Ginseng, Korean White (*Panax ginseng*, dried root). Considered stronger than Siberian Ginseng, but weaker than Woodsgrown American or Wild American Ginseng. Has the same properties and is used for the same conditions as Wild American Ginseng.

Dose: *Take 15-25 drops in morning and afternoon. Best to pulse (see pages 28 & 49).*

Ginseng, Siberian (*Eleutherococcus senticosus*, dried root). Not a true "Panax" Ginseng as with the other Ginsengs listed here, but has very similar actions. This Ginseng works more slowly but it can be taken for extended periods of time. As an adaptogen (i.e., a substance which produces a normalizing effect on the body), it increases strength, endurance, and resistance to stress or infection. Useful for those who have decreased resistance due to stimulant, alcohol and drug use. Also helpful for those who thrive on stress (type A personalities).
Dose: Take 20 drops three times a day.

Ginseng, Wild American (*Panax quinquefolium*, dried white root). Considered the highest quality "white" Ginseng. For emotional and physical stress manifesting as elevated blood sugar (triglycerides) and blood lipids (cholesterol), exhaustion and depression. Use when recuperating from illness or surgery. As an excellent adaptogen (i.e., a substance which produces a normalizing effect on the body), it increases strength, endurance, and resistance to stress or infection.
Dose: Take 10-25 drops in late afternoon. Best to pulse (see pages 28 & 49).

Ginseng, Woodsgrown American (*Panax quinquefolium*, dried white root). Used for the same conditions as indicated under Wild American Ginseng. The difference between Woodsgrown American Ginseng and Wild American Ginseng is that Woodsgrown American Ginseng is considered a medium quality Ginseng because it is cultivated domestically for one year and then transplanted into the forest; whereas Wild American Ginseng sprouts from seed already present in the forest environment. Chinese connoisseurs value both Ginsengs but Wild American Ginseng is more prized and fetches higher prices.
Dose: Take 15-30 drops in late afternoon. Best to pulse (see pages 28 & 49).

Golden Seal (*Hydrastis canadensis*, dried root). Use

WERNEKE © 1993

American Ginseng

for sub-acute or chronic mucous membrane inflammation occurring in sinusitis, hay fever, allergies, gastritis, stomach ulcers, colitis, diarrhea, sore gums and throat, or tonsillitis.
Dose: *Take 10-25 drops up to five times a day. Use only until the inflammatory stage goes away, then discontinue use. Not for long term use. Do not exceed recommended dose. Best to pulse (see pages 28 & 49).*
Contraindications: *Not in pregnancy.*

Golden Seal/Echinacea Complex™ A favorite for fighting a cold or flu. Reduces inflammation and strengthens tissues of the throat, sinuses and bronchioles. Liquifies mucus, relieves deep-seated joint, muscle and bone pains, and headaches, as well as generalized body aches and headaches. Breaks fevers and stimulates the immune system's response. Quickly eliminates waste products and helps the body regain its balance.
Dose: *If symptoms are acute, take 20-30 drops every hour. For other indications, take 20-30 drops three to four times a day. Best to pulse (see pages 28 & 49).*
Contraindications: *Not in pregnancy.*
Ingredients: *Golden Seal, Echinacea, Elderberry, Licorice, Yerba Mansa, Yarrow, Elder blossom, Boneset, Bayberry, Dandelion, Ginger, Grindelia, Red Root, Osha.*

Gotu Kola (*Centella asiatica*, fresh herb). Enhances memory, clarity and calmness. Great support for the thyroid gland when low function contributes to emotional depression, dry skin, cold extremities, poor digestion, weight gain and/or little endurance. Use also for eczema, psoriasis and varicose veins.
Dose: *Take 20-30 drops morning and mid-afternoon. Best to pulse (see pages 28 & 49).*

Gravel Root (*Eupatorium purpureum*, dried root). Use for bladder or prostate irritation with urgent, difficult and frequent urination, cystitis, nephritis or urethritis. Helps prevent formation of kidney stones.
Dose: *Take 20-60 drops twice a day. Best to pulse (see pages 28 & 49).*
Contraindications: *Do not use in pregnancy or while nursing.*

Hawthorn (*Crataegus spp.*, fresh flower and berry). For heart irregularities with rapid heart beat episodes or weakness of heart muscle from poor blood supply. Prevents complications in almost all heart diseases, especially angina and congestive heart failure.

Note: *Not useful for damaged heart where the damage is termed organic. Works best for functional heart problems (i.e., angina).*

Dose: *Take 10-20 drops up to three times a day for one month, then twice a day for an unlimited period of time.*

Hawthorn/Motherwort Complex (see Cardiotonic™)

HB Pressure Tonic™ (Linden/Hawthorn Complex). Helpful in cases of mild to moderately elevated blood pressure. Especially helpful when high blood pressure is due to stress or is aggravated by excessive sodium intake. Useful in either systolic or diastolic elevations.

Dose: *Take 20-40 drops two or three times a day.*

Contraindications: *Not in pregnancy.*

Side effects: *High dosages may lead to excessively low blood pressure. Continue to monitor your blood pressure to make sure herbal treatment is working for you.*

Ingredients: *Linden flowers, Mistletoe, Dandelion, Passion Flower, Hawthorn flower and berry, Siberian Ginseng, Yarrow, Skullcap, Prickly Ash bark.*

Hearty Hawthorn (see Cardiotonic™)

Herbaprofen™ (Jamaican Dogwood/Black Cohosh Complex). A good muscular anti-spasmodic and anti-inflammatory formula. As a botanical analgesic, it helps reduce pain and spasms caused by toothaches, uterine and fallopian cramps, neuralgia, intestinal colic, gallstones and renal colics, rheumatoid arthritis, fibrositis, sore muscles, spasmodic cough, sciatica, sprained back, etc. Useful for congestive headaches. Especially beneficial where pain prevents sleep.

Dose: *Take 20-50 drops up to every three hours, or as needed. Best to pulse (see pages 28 & 49).*

Contraindications: *Not in pregnancy or while nursing.*

Ingredients: *Jamaican Dogwood, Black Cohosh, Wood Betony, Meadowsweet, Kava Kava, Passion Flower, Devil's Claw, Licorice, Stevia.*

Hops (*Humulus lupulus*, dry strobile). For insomnia caused by heartburn, indigestion, restlessness and/or headaches. Calms hyper-secretion of stomach acids while toning up stomach muscles and digestive functions.

Dose: *Take 10-40 drops three times a day. Best to pulse*

(see pages 28 & 49).
Contraindications: *Not during depression.*
Side effects: *Long term use may cause depression.*

Horse Chestnut/Witch Hazel Complex (see Vein Tonic™)

Horsetail (*Equisetum arvense*, fresh Spring-gathered herb). Stops slow oozing bleeding of all kinds. Useful for children who wet the bed. Useful with connective tissue weaknesses as may be found in kidneys, lungs and liver. High in silica. Stimulates calcium absorption. Useful in arthritis.
Dose: *Take 15-30 drops up to three times a day. For bed wetting in children over five years old, use with California Poppy, 10 drops of each twice a day. Best to pulse (see pages 28 & 49).*

Hyssop (*Hyssopus officinalis*, fresh herb). For lung problems characterized by excess mucus production with difficult expectoration. Useful for coughs, bronchitis, asthma, chronic mucus, gas, and stomach irritation.
Dose: *Take 10-40 drops up to four times a day. Best to pulse (see pages 28 & 49).*

Ivy Itch ReLeaf™ (Jewelweed/Plantain Complex) FOR EXTERNAL USE ONLY. Stimulates maximum healing power in the case of poison ivy or poison oak dermatitis. May also be used for herpes outbreaks (mouth or genital). Offers relief in cases of insect stings and bites, as well as rashes caused by stinging nettles. Use on impetigo, skin rashes, eczema, psoriasis and other dermatitis.
Dose: *Spray liberally on affected areas every two hours. Let dry. Best to pulse (see pages 28 & 49).*
Ingredients: *Jewelweed, Grindelia, Plantain, Licorice, Echinacea.*

Jamaican Dogwood/Black Cohosh Complex (see Herbaprofen™)

Jewelweed/Plaintain Complex (see Ivy Itch ReLeaf™)

Juniper Berries (*Juniperus communis*, dried berry). Useful as an antiseptic in sub-acute or chronic inflammation of the bladder or urethra, i.e., the kind of inflammation that has been there for a while and has not healed properly. Also for chronic arthritis, gout and rheumatism.
Dose: *Take 15-30 drops three times a day. Do not take*

for more than six weeks in succession. Best to pulse (see pages 28 & 49).

Contraindications: *Not in pregnancy. Not in acute urinary tract infection, stomach inflammation or serious kidney disease.*

Side effects: *May aggravate inflammation.*

Kava Kava (*Piper methysticum*, dried root). Useful in relieving nervousness, agitation, tension, stress and anxiety. Kava Kava is a mood elevator, and although it is slightly stimulating, it helps relax muscle tension due to stress, relieves fatigue and calms the mind. It is very useful when anxiety prevents sleep.

Dose: *Take 20-30 drops two to three times a day. Best to pulse (see pages 28 & 49).*

Kidalin™ (Catnip/Kola Complex). Specific for Attention Deficit Disorder (ADD) also known as Attention Deficit Hyperactivity Disorder (ADHD). Reduces aggressiveness, focuses and relaxes the mind, rebuilds the nervous system and calms the hyperkinetic behavior in those with ADHD. Lessens symptoms such as short attention span, jitteriness, restlessness, difficulty concentrating, constant shifting and fretting, difficulty completing assigned tasks, excessive running, climbing and talking. Also helpful if symptoms manifest as an inability to focus and pay attention without symptoms of overactivity or impulsivity.

Dose: *Syrup for children five to nine years old, take one half teaspoon every four hours. Syrup for children ten years old and older, take one teaspoon twice a day. Extract for adults, take 20-40 drops two to three times a day. Best to pulse (see pages 28 & 49) by taking five days on and two days off.*

Contraindications: *Not in pregnancy.*

Ingredients: *Catnip, Damiana, Kola nut, Lavender, Chamomile, Periwinkle, Lemon Balm, Licorice, Oat seeds. Comes in natural and three flavors.*

Kidney Tonic™ (Dandelion/Uva Ursi Complex). For non-specific inflammation of the kidneys or bladder, lower back pain, water retention in PMS or from changes in heat or humidity. Use in low grade bacterial infection of the urethra or bladder and irritation of the urethra after sex. It is specific for women who get recurrent urinary tract infections after sex. Used over a period of time, it will strengthen the urinary system.

Dose: *For acute problems take 20-30 drops every four hours. As a preventative, take 15 drops twice a day. Best to pulse (see pages 28 & 49).*

Contraindications: *Not in pregnancy.*

Side effects: *Urine may have a peculiar smell and color.*

Ingredients: *Dandelion, Saw Palmetto, Parsley root, Couch grass, Boldo, Buchu, Juniper berries, Uva Ursi, Pipsissewa, Cubeb berries.*

Korean White Ginseng (see Ginseng, Korean White)

Kudzu (*Pueraria lobata*, dried root and flowers). Used in Traditional Chinese Medicine to treat the effects of alcohol drunkenness or hangovers. Also used for skin rashes. Researchers have concluded that Kudzu helps decrease desire for alcohol and may help in migraine headaches, neck stiffness and hypertension.

Dose: *Take 20-40 drops three to five times a day. Best to pulse (see pages 28 & 49).*

Licorice (*Glycyrrhiza uralensis*, dried root). Effective adrenal gland support. For gastric ulcers, bronchial spasms, sore throats, painful menstruation, arthritis or herpes. Offers support in AIDS as research suggests it may inhibit the virus. Also has mild anti-inflammatory, anti-histaminic and laxative properties.

Dose: *Take 20-30 drops up to three times a day. Best to pulse (see pages 28 & 49).*

Contraindications: *Not in pregnancy or when high blood pressure from sodium retention is present.*

Side effects: *Large amounts may cause sodium retention, leading to high blood pressure.*

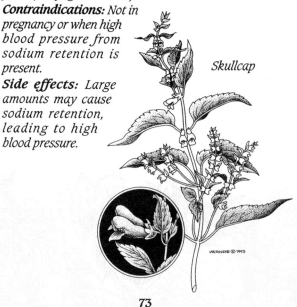

Skullcap

WERNEKE © 1993

Linden/Hawthorn Complex
(see HB Pressure Tonic™)

Liver Tonic™ (Milk Thistle/Oregon Grape Complex). Protects and repairs the liver. Relieves liver and gall bladder pain which may occur after excessive ingestion of fatty foods, alcohol, coffee and chocolate. Should be taken by people exposed to aromatic hydrocarbons, solvents, paints, thinners, etc. Use when there are elevated liver enzymes (SGOT, SGPT), difficulty digesting fats, or during hepatitis flare-ups. Also for mild frontal headaches after fatty meals, for mild constipation and simple jaundice. Finally, it lowers high bilirubin levels.
Dose: *Take 15-25 drops three times a day. Best to pulse (see pages 28 & 49).*
Contraindications: *Not in pregnancy.*
Ingredients: *Milk Thistle, Toadflax, Oregon Grape root, Echinacea, Licorice, Greater Celandine, Fringetree bark, Culver's root, Blue Flag.*

Lobelia (*Lobelia inflata*, dried plant in the bladder seed stage). Specific for bronchial spasms as may occur in asthma. Helps decrease craving for nicotine when quitting smoking.
Dose: *Take 5-20 drops not more than three times a day. Do not exceed recommended dosage. Best to pulse (see pages 28 & 49).*
Contraindications: *Not in pregnancy.*
Side effects: *May cause nausea and vomiting. Excessive amount slows heart beat and depresses respiration.*

Lobelia/Oat Seeds Complex
(see Smoke Free Drops™)

Lomatium (*Lomatium dissectum*, dried root). Used for lung problems, pneumonia, flu and fevers. Lomatium shortens the duration of respiratory viral infections. Very helpful with Chronic Fatigue Immuno-Deficiency Syndrome, Epstein-Barr virus and cytomegalovirus infection.
Dose: *Take 15-30 drops up to four times a day. Best to pulse (see pages 28 & 49).*
Contraindications: *Do not take in combination with blood thinning agents.*
Side effects: *Skin rash. If rash occurs, discontinue extract and rash will promptly disappear.*

Lung Tonic™ (Mullein/Horehound Complex). Specific support for Chronic Obstructive Pulmonary Disease (COPD), including emphysema, chronic bronchitis and asthma. Useful for congestion, inflammation of bronchioles and lung tissue, spasms of bronchioles and excessive production of mucus. Helps protect against respiratory infection, soothes and calms coughs. Ideal formula for long-term management of lung problems.

Dose: *Take 20-30 drops three times a day (mid-morning, mid-afternoon, and early evening), for an unlimited period of time.*

Ingredients: *Mullein, Horehound, Elecampane, Grindelia, Echinacea, Pleurisy Root, Passion Flower, Osha, Lobelia, Yerba Santa.*

Lymphatonic™ (Echinacea/Red Root Complex). Excellent deep acting immune system cleaner. A must for recurring or lingering, hard to shake colds, flu, infections and frequent minor illnesses. Use for acute swelling of tonsils and/or lymph nodes. Specific for uterine, ovarian or breast cysts. Speeds up healing of cuts, boils, or other poorly healing abrasions. Useful to shorten healing time of poison ivy or poison oak infection as well as cat-scratch disease.

Dose: *For acute symptoms, take 15-25 drops every hour. In chronic stage, take 25-40 drops two to three times day. Best to pulse (see pages 28 & 49). For cysts, take with Red Root, 20 drops of each three times a day.*

Contraindications: *Not in pregnancy*

Ingredients: *Echinacea, Red Root, Ocotillo, Burdock, Licorice, Dandelion, Yellow Dock, Wild Indigo, Blue Flag, Stillingia.*

Ma Huang (see Ephedra)

Ma Huang/Mullein Complex (see Decongestonic™)

Ma Huang/Yerba Mansa Complex (see Congest Free™)

Marshmallow (*Althaea officinalis*, fresh root). For any inflammation of the digestive system, such as the mouth, stomach, intestines and colon. Also soothes sore throats.

Dose: *Take 20-40 drops up to five times a day.*

Meadowsweet (*Filipendula ulmaria*, dried pre-flowering herb). Aspirin substitute. For inflammation of muscles or joints, rheumatic, arthritic and gout. Offers relief in heart-

burn, hyperacidity, nausea, cystitis, nephritis, menstrual cramps, gastritis and peptic ulcers. Helps in reducing fevers.
Dose: *Take 15-25 drops up to four times a day. Best to pulse (see pages 28 & 49).*

Menopautonic™ (Dong Quai/Vitex Complex). Decreases or stops menopausal symptoms such as hot flashes, sweating, nervousness, insomnia, urinary frequency and back pain. Normalizes the menstrual cycle of women who have discontinued use of oral contraceptives, or those who are having erratic cycles (excessively long or short). Lifts menopausal depression within a week.
Dose: *Take 20-30 drops early morning and before retiring.*
Contraindications: *Not in pregnancy.*
Ingredients: *Dong Quai, Vitex, Hawthorn flowers, Black Cohosh, False Unicorn Root, Motherwort, Licorice, Passion Flower, Siberian Ginseng, Pipsissewa, Woodsgrown American Ginseng, Dulse.*

Menotime™ (see Menopautonic™)

Migra Free™ (Feverfew/Periwinkle Complex). Migra Free contains a guaranteed potency of 400 mcg of Parthenolide per ml, the amount proven effective in clinical trials to stop migraine headache attacks. A truly wonderful preventative formula. Taken every day, it prevents inflammation of blood vessels in the brain and stops migraine headaches before they begin, even those headache attacks resistant to conventional medicines.

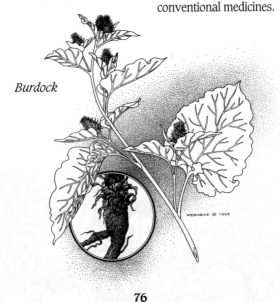

Burdock

WERNEKE © 1995

Dose: *During an acute migraine attack, take 40 drops every hour until migraine subsides. As a preventative, take 40 drops once a day. Can be taken for an unlimited period of time.*

Ingredients: *Feverfew, Periwinkle, Ginkgo, Meadowsweet, White Willow, Stevia.*

Milk Thistle (*Silybum marianum*, dried seed). The premier liver herb! Useful for chronic hepatitis, for fatty livers of alcoholics or even for cirrhosis of the liver. Protects the liver from harmful substances such as alcohol, fumes, and drugs, and stimulates its regeneration. Protects individuals who may come in long-term contact with chemicals, metals or aromatic hydrocarbons, such as solvents.

Dose: *Take 10-25 drops up to three times a day.*

Milk Thistle Complex (see Liver Tonic™)

Milk Thistle/Oregon Grape Complex (see Liver Tonic™)

Montezuma's ReLeaf™ (Sweet Annie/Quassia Complex*).* Prevents and counters amoebic, giardial or other types of parasitic infections where infection produces intestinal gas, diarrhea and mild to severe abdominal cramps. A must when traveling in foreign countries. Use when there is pain in the lower right abdomen, dull twinges with constipation or diarrhea, and poor fat digestion and absorption.

Dose: *Against infection, take 15-30 drops every two to three hours. As a preventative, take 10 drops ten minutes before each meal.*

Contraindications: *Not in pregnancy.*

Ingredients: *Sweet Annie, Quassia, Oregon Grape Root, Bistort, Ginger, Angelica, Bayberry.*

Motherwort (*Leonorus cardiaca*, fresh flowering herb). Reduces water retention and menstrual cramps. Decreases the amount, length and severity of hot flashes and menopausal depression. Restores elasticity and thickness of post-menopausal vaginal walls. Also excellent for calming rapid heart beat, palpitation and hypertension from thyroid stress.

Dose: *Take 20-50 drops up to four times a day. Best to pulse (see pages 28 & 49).*

Contraindications: *Not in pregnancy.*

Mouth Tonic™ (Myrrh/Golden Seal Complex). Used primarily as an external treatment for mouth and gum sores, bleeding gums, fever blisters, herpes sores and mouth ulcers (aphtous stomatitis), sores from dentures, enlarged and spongy tonsils and receding gums due to degeneration. Wonderful for pyorrhea and periodontal disease. May be taken internally for colds and flu.

Dose: Apply with cotton swab twice a day. Do not rinse. If stinging or irritation occurs, dilute with a little water. Internally: 20-30 drops every two to three hours.

Ingredients: Echinacea, Myrrh, Golden Seal, Propolis, Yerba Mansa, Bloodroot.

M-Roid ReLeaf™ (Butcher's Broom/Collinsonia Complex). Useful for hemorrhoids, varicocele, prostatitis, urethritis, bladder irritation and acute bowel disorders, especially when there is a sense of constriction, pain and irritation in the pelvic area. This formula increases blood supply system drainage from the intestines, prostate and pelvic areas and relieves liver congestion (portal circulation congestion).

Dose: Best to pulse (see pages 28 & 49) by taking 20-30 drops twice a day for three weeks. Stop for one week. Repeat.

Contraindications: Not in pregnancy.

Ingredients: Butcher's Broom, Collinsonia, Horse Chestnut, Ocotillo, Red Root, Milk Thistle, Yellow Dock, Bog Bean, Yarrow, Licorice, Stevia.

Mullein (*Verbascum thapsus*, fresh top leaf). Specific for coughs, especially in older asthmatic patients. Very useful for sub-acute or chronic bronchitis, emphysema or Chronic Obstructive Pulmonary Disease which worsens with nervousness.

Dose: Take 25-40 drops every three hours. Best to pulse (see pages 28 & 49).

Mullein/Horehound Complex (see Lung Tonic™)

Mullein/Garlic Ear Drops™ FOR EXTERNAL USE ONLY. Specific to prevent or reduce middle ear infection (Otitis media). Acts as a gentle bacteriostatic, helps to reduce pain and assists in establishing the proper acidity/alkalinity ratio of the ear area.

Dose and usage directions: Warm the oil to body temperature, put 1-4 drops in each ear, insert sterile cotton in each ear to prevent dripping. Repeat every six to eight hours.

Contraindications: *Do not use in ears with perforated eardrums.*

Ingredients: *Mullein flower, Garlic (fresh cloves and oil), in a base of olive oil and vitamin E.*

Myrrh (*Commiphora myrrha*, gum exudate). For painful ulceration of the gums or mouth as in herpes or gingivitis, pharyngitis, sinusitis, laryngitis and indigestion. Taken in combination with Echinacea, Myrrh helps to elevate low white blood cell level.

Dose: *Take 10-20 drops four times a day. Best to pulse (see pages 28 & 49).*

Contraindications: *Not in pregnancy or in overt kidney disease.*

Myrrh/Golden Seal Complex (see Mouth Tonic™)

Nervine Tonic™ (Passion Flower/Valerian Complex). An excellent all purpose daily sedative. Useful for soothing muscle twitches, nervousness, anxiety, nervous-type asthma, muscle pain or tightness from stress or overexertion, intestinal cramps, exhaustion. Also helps while breaking the cycle of drug addiction. Good herbal remedy to take the edge off pain. It decreases irritability of the nervous system and gently stimulates its repair.

Dose: *Take 15-50 drops every three or four hours. Best to pulse (see pages 28 & 49).*

Contraindications: *Not in pregnancy.*

Ingredients: *Passion Flower, Valerian root, Oat seeds, Black Cohosh, Skullcap, Betony.*

Nettle (*Urtica dioica*, fresh herb). Specific for hay fever and allergic rhinitis. Also for vaginitis, rheumatoid arthritis, stomatitis, eczema, diarrhea, hemorrhoids, asthma and gout. Tones up the mucous membranes especially where excessive mucus and inflammation are present. An alkalizing diuretic.

Dose: *For acute hay fever, 20 drops every half to one hour. In other cases, 15-20 drops three times a day.*

Nettle/Eyebright Complex (see Allertonic™)

Oat Seeds (*Avena sativa*, fresh seed in the milky stage). One of the best nervous system tonics available. Excellent for recuperating from a stressful experience or after an emotional breakdown. Helps in the withdrawal of nicotine, cocaine or opiates.

Dose: *Take 25 drops three times a day. Take for at least one month or more to achieve best results.*

Oats/Damiana Complex (see Passion Potion™)

Osha (*Ligusticum porteri*, dried root). A great herb at the beginning of a cold or flu. For early stages of: sore throat, chest cold with painful breathing, thick stringy mucus, or dry asthma. Stimulates the immune system and prevents secondary infections. Prevents recurrent middle ear infection in children; loosens and expels mucus.

Dose: *Take 20-40 drops three to four times a day. Best to pulse (see pages 28 & 49).*

Contraindications: *Not in pregnancy.*

Osha/Pleurisy Root Complex (see Respiratonic™)

Osha Root Complex Syrup™ Stops or calms cough. Decreases lung congestion, promotes expectoration, and reduces inflammation of throat and bronchioles. Soothes and slightly anesthetizes the throat.

Dose: *Take 1/2 to 1 teaspoon every three to four hours. Children, two to five years old, take 1/4 to 1/2 teaspoon every three to four hours. Best to pulse (see pages 28 & 49).*

Contraindications: *Not during the first three months of pregnancy.*

Ingredients: *Osha, Wild Cherry bark, White Pine bark, Balm of Gilead, Spikenard, and Bloodroot in a* glycerine/gum arabic syrup base.

Para-Free™ (Black Walnut/Wormwood Complex). This formula is designed to eliminate parasites such as giardia, entamoeba and other protozoal bugs. It inhibits pinworms and other types of parasites and tones up the digestive system.

Dose: *Take 40 drops twice a day before meals. Best to pulse (see pages 28 & 49).*

Contraindications: *Not in pregnancy or while nursing.*

Ingredients: *Fresh "green" Black Walnut hulls, Wormwood, Quassia, Cloves, Male Fern.*

Passion Flower (*Passiflora incarnata*, fresh flowering herb). For the "chattering" brain which prevents sleep. Calms the mind in headstrong individuals. Good for menopausal nervousness and anxiety, for persistent hiccough, and for frequent asthma attacks in children.

Dose: *For adults, 20-40 drops up to four times a day. For children five years and older, 10 drops up to four times a day.*

Passion Flower/Valerian Complex (see Nervine Tonic™)

Passion Potion™ (Oats/Damiana {T. aphrodisiaca} Complex). Taken over time, an excellent sexual tonic for both men and women as it builds deep energy reserves. As a general tonic, Passion Potion™ reinstates a sense of passion back in life and stimulates a feeling of "well being." Specific for exhaustion, mild depression, chronic anxiety states, and/or during convalescence or any state of debility. Taken over time, increases stamina, decreases outbreaks of herpes and shingles, enhances one's vitality and tones the central nervous system. As a prelude to making love, it relaxes the mind and opens the heart.

Dose: *Take 20-40 drops twice a day. If using for the longer term health issues as noted above, take for at least one month or more to achieve best results.*

Ingredients: *Oat seeds, Damiana, Passion Flower, Hawthorn flowers, leaves and berries, Woodsgrown American Ginseng, Licorice, Nettle, Stevia, Parsley root.*

Pau D'Arco (*Tabebuia impetiginosa*, Argentinian dried inner bark). Internally: Take for systemic candida infections, and fungal infections of the mouth (thrush). Externally: Use for fungal infection in feet, babies' fannies or women's vaginas.

Dose: *Internally: Take 15-25 drops up to four times a day. Best to pulse (see pages 28 & 49). Externally: Dilute with a little water and apply.*

Note: *For babies less than six months old, use EXTERNALLY only.*

Pau D'Arco/Black Walnut Complex (see Yeast ReLeaf™)

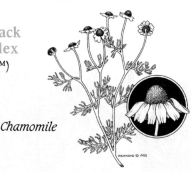

Chamomile

Pennyroyal (*Hedeoma pulegioides*, fresh pre-flowering herb). Specific for late, painful, spotty menstruation accompanied by sore breasts, bloating, and other PMS symptoms. Helps to induce delayed menstruation. Helps to break dry fever, calms coughs and stimulates mucus expectoration.

Dose: *Take 20-40 drops in water three to four times a day. Best to pulse (see pages 28 & 49). To stimulate sweating, take in hot water.*

Contraindications: *Not in pregnancy.*

Peppermint (*Mentha piperita*, fresh pre-flowering herb). Stops nausea or vomiting. Stimulates the production and release of bile; prevents intestinal fermentation; stops gas formation and stomach and intestinal cramping.

Dose: *Take 10-20 drops after meals.*

Pipsissewa (*Chimaphila umbellata*, fresh herb). For bladder, kidney or urethra irritation or infection, especially after overindulging in alkaline foods, fruits and vegetables. Also for prostate irritation when dull pain occurs upon first urination in morning.

Dose: *Take 10-25 drops up to four times a day Best to pulse (see pages 28 & 49).*

Pleurisy Root (*Asclepias tuberosa*, dried root). As its name implies, useful in pleurisy, pneumonia, bronchitis or chest colds with dry respiratory membranes and skin. For dry skin problems, such as eczema or psoriasis.

Dose: *Take 15-30 drops three to four times a day. Best to pulse (see pages 28 & 49).*

Contraindications: *Not in pregnancy.*

Side effects: *Excessive amounts may cause nausea and vomiting.*

PMS ReLeaf™ (Vitex/Dandelion Complex). Stabilizes the emotional and physical components of PMS. Eliminates excess fluids; supports the liver; prevents build up of prostaglandins; stimulates fluid drainage from congested tissues (breasts and pelvic area). Reduces PMS symptoms such as water retention, swollen and tender breasts, lower backache, cramping, fatigue, irritability, insomnia, depression, difficulty in concentrating, panic attacks, anxiety, mood swings, crying, physical and emotional tension, low blood sugar, low sex drive, headaches and migraines.

Dose: *For acute symptoms, take 30 drops every three to* *four hours as needed. For chronic conditions or extreme PMS symptoms, take 30 drops three times a day beginning up to two weeks prior to menstruation. Also consider taking Cycle 1 Estrotonic™ and Cycle 2 Progestonic™. For painful cramping, also consider taking Cramp ReLeaf™ or Herbaprofen™.*

Contraindications: *Not in pregnancy.*

Ingredients: *Vitex, Dandelion, Fringetree, Nettle, Red Root, Western Pasque Flower, Cramp Bark, Cleavers, Ginger, Stevia.*

Propolis (Dry gum from beehives). For mouth, gum and intestinal infections; foul smelling diarrhea from intestinal infections. For skin abrasions, especially in moist areas such as feet, hands and face.

Dose: *Internally: Take 15-30 drops up to four times a day. Best to pulse (see pages 28 & 49). Externally: Dilute and apply.*

Contraindications: *Should not be used internally by those with known reactions to bees or bee products, such as bee pollen or honey.*

Prostatonic™ (Saw Palmetto/Damiana Complex). Offers relief for benign enlargement of the prostate when enlargement has caused varying degrees of urinary problems such as frequent and urgent urination, difficulty in urinating or sensation of incomplete emptying of the bladder and dribbling. Helps reduce inflammation of these tissues and increases uptake of circulating male hormones. Also soothes genital pain caused by excessive sexual activity.

Dose: *Take 20-30 drops two to three times a day for an unlimited period of time. It may take up to six weeks for effects to be realized.*

Ingredients: *Saw Palmetto, Nettle root, Yarrow, Dong Quai, Woodsgrown American Ginseng, Cleavers, Yerba Mansa, Sarsaparilla, Damiana, Kava Kava.*

Red Clover (*Trifolium pratense*, fresh flower). High in minerals. Good as a maintenance liquid during infections, hepatitis or mononucleosis. Helps increase lactation in nursing mothers. Also helpful for psoriasis and eczema.

Dose: *Take 15-30 drops up to four times a day. Dosage for children: 10 drops up to four times a day.*

Red Clover/Burdock Complex (see Dermatonic™)

Red Ginseng/Fo-ti Complex (see Bionic Tonic™)

Red Raspberry (*Rubus idaeus*, fresh leaf). Used in pregnancy to prevent spotting during the first trimester and to increase overall muscle tone of the uterine walls. Also for excessive menstrual bleeding and mild diarrhea. Use diluted as a rinse for mouth ulcers and bleeding gums.

Dose: *Internally: Take 15-30 drops up to three times a day. Externally: Use diluted as a wash.*

Red Root (*Ceanothus americanus*, dried root). For acute tonsillitis or sore throat; inflamed spleen and/or inflamed lymphatic nodes, and fluid cysts in breasts, ovaries, uterus or testes.

Dose: *Take 20-40 drops up to four times a day. Best to pulse (see pages 28 & 49). For cysts, take with Lymphatonic™, 20 drops of each three times a day.*

Contraindications: *Not during coagulation therapies or if serious blood disorders are present.*

Remember Now™ (Ginkgo/Gotu Kola Complex). Specific for memory disorders, poor concentration and symptoms of primary cerebral arteriosclerosis, such as poor memory, irritability, restlessness, speech and motor (movement) disorders, vertigo, headaches and lack of attention. Has a positive effect on tinnitus, dizziness and hearing defects, especially when these occur in old age because of poor blood circulation. Also very useful after strokes.

Dose: *Take 20-30 drops two times a day for an unlimited period of time. May take up to six weeks for effects to be felt.*

Ingredients: *Ginkgo, Periwinkle, Gotu Kola, Peppermint, Oat seeds, St. John's Wort, Siberian Ginseng, Rosemary, Prickly Ash bark.*

Respiratonic™ (Osha/Pleurisy Root Complex). Relieves chest colds, lung congestion, acute bronchitis and pleurisy. All-purpose expectorant which loosens mucus, dilates the bronchioles and stimulates general resistance. Decreases excessive heat in the lungs, eases pain of coughing and liquifies mucus.

Dose: *Take 10-25 drops every two to three hours. Best to pulse (see pages 28 & 49).*

Contraindications: *Not in pregnancy.*

Ingredients: *Echinacea, Osha, Licorice, Yerba Mansa, Yerba Santa, Pleurisy Root, Grindelia, Ginger.*

Sarsaparilla (*Smilax spp.*, dried root). Useful in simple prostate enlargement. Increases elimination of urea and uric acid. Helpful in gout, herpes, many types of skin problems, rheumatism and sores. For moderate deficiencies of adrenal or gonad hormonal production.
Dose: *Take 15-20 drops three times a day.*

Saw Palmetto (*Serenoa repens*, semi-dried berry). Specific for simple prostate enlargement. For difficulty urinating, especially with benign prostatic hypertrophy and dribbling of urine. Useful when reproductive glands are tender from excessive sexual activity.
Dose: *Take 20-30 drops up to four times a day for an unlimited period of time. It may take up to six weeks for effects to kick in.*

Saw Palmetto/Damiana Complex
(see Prostatonic™)

Schisandra (*Schisandra chinensis [Wu Wei Zi]*, dried berries). Increases overall resistance. Helps fight stress, fatigue, tiredness, exhaustion and depression. Helps in allergic skin disorders. Considered nearly as good a general tonic as Ginseng.
Dose: *Take 15-25 drops twice a day for at least 100 days to achieve best results.*

7 Ginsengs™ The ultimate Ginseng tonic. Most complete, well rounded rejuvenating product available. Excellent for emotional or physical exhaustion, as a tonic after a prolonged illness or in depression from major neurological or autoimmune disease. A great extract to help prepare for or recuperate from major stress. Best adaptogenic formula to support and enhance your well being.
Dose: *Take 10-25 drops twice a day for at least one month to achieve best results.*

Golden Seal

WERNEKE © 1993

Ingredients: *Wild American Ginseng, Woodsgrown American Ginseng, Kirin Chinese Red Ginseng, Shui-Chu Chinese Red Ginseng, Korean White Ginseng, Cultivated American Ginseng, Siberian Ginseng.*

Sheep Sorrel/Burdock Complex (see Essiac Tonic™)

Shepherd's Purse (*Capsella bursa-pastoris*, fresh herb). For excessive uterine bleeding or bleeding hemorrhoids. Specific for acute attacks of gout or any other conditions in which blood uric acid is elevated.
Dose: *Take 15-30 drops three times a day. For acute gout attack, take 30 drops every two hours for a day or two. Best to pulse (see pages 28 & 49).*
Contraindications: *Not in pregnancy.*
Warning: *If prolonged, significant or unusual bleeding occurs, seek medical attention.*

Siberian Ginseng (see Ginseng, Siberian)

Siberian Ginseng/Devil's Claw Complex (see Cholesterotonic™)

Singer's Saving Grace™ (Collinsonia/Jack-in-the-Pulpit Complex*)*. Ideal for sore throats, laryngitis, pharyngitis, hoarseness, cough, expectoration of thick mucus and a feeling of dryness in the throat. A blessing for singers, preachers, teachers or anybody with a sore throat from singing, screaming, cheering, shouting or talking loudly for a long period of time. Also for sore throats at the beginning of a cold or as an aftermath of a lung infection.
Dose: *Spray two or three times directly into the mouth every one to four hours.*
Ingredients: *Yerba Mansa, Collinsonia, Licorice, Jack-in-the-Pulpit, Osha, Propolis, Echinacea, Ginger.*

Skullcap (*Scutellaria lateriflora*, fresh flowering herb). For inability to sleep, edgy feelings, restlessness, phantom pains after amputation, muscle twitching, neuralgia, pain from shingles, and sciatica.
Dose: *Take 20-40 drops up to four times a day. Best to pulse (see pages 28 & 49).*

Slippery Elm (*Ulmus fulva*, dried inner bark). Useful for gastritis, enteritis, colitis, mouth and throat inflammation, duodenal ulcers, and diarrhea.
Dose: *Take 10-30 drops up to five times a day.*

Smoke Free Drops™ (Lobelia/Oat Seeds Complex). Ideal herbal combination formula for those wishing to stop smoking. Decreases withdrawal symptoms, calms the nervous system, dilates the bronchioles and loosens mucus. It is not habit forming and greatly assists the determined person who wishes to stop smoking.

Dose: *Take 20-30 drops every two to three hours.*
Contraindications: *Not in pregnancy.*
Ingredients: *Lobelia, Oat seeds, Licorice, Osha, Passion Flower, Pleurisy Root, Grindelia, Mullein, Ginger.*

St. John's Wort (*Hypericum perforatum*, fresh and dry pre-flowering herb). Effective for depression, anxiety, agitation, insomnia, loss of interest, and excessive sleeping. Used to treat retro-viral infections such as HIV and AIDS (this last indication is still under investigation).

Dose: *Take 15-40 drops three times a day. Must be taken for at least three months to impact depression.*

Contraindications: *Fair-skinned individuals should avoid excessive exposure to sunlight while on St. John's Wort, since this herb may cause increased photo-sensitivity.*

St. John's Wort/Lemon Balm Complex
(see Deprezac™)

Stomach Tonic™ (Chamomile/Catnip Complex). Offers immediate relief for bloating, gas cramps, pain after eating, stomach acidity, and helps to soothe pain of stomach ulcers. Sweetens the breath and dispels nausea and vomiting. For ulcerated stomach, take Stomach Tonic™ to ease pain and symptoms between meals and during the night. Use Digestonic™ before meals to tone and regulate the flow of stomach digestive juices.

Dose: *For adults, take 5-15 drops in a little water three times a day, after meals or before bedtime. For babies, give 1-2 drops, diluted in a liquid, up to three times a day, after meals or before bedtime.*
Note: *Safe for babies two months and older.*
Contraindications: *Not in pregnancy.*
Ingredients: *Chamomile, Catnip, Fennel, Lavender, Star Anise, Cardamom, Gentian, Angelica, Prickly Ash berry.*

Stone Root (See Collinsonia)

Sweet Annie/Quassia Complex (see Montezuma's ReLeaf™)

Triple Source Echinacea™ A complete spectrum, full-potency Echinacea formula rooted in native North American traditional medicine, and in cutting edge European Phytopharmaceutical research. As a first line immune system activator, it is ideal for the initial stages of colds and at the beginning of a general infection. Stimulates production, maturation, mobilization and aggressiveness of white blood cells and other body defenses against intruders. Prevents or slows down bacterial and viral infections by strengthening the connective tissues. Helps boost the immune system prior to cold and flu season. Helps reduce swelling and stimulates repair in tendonitis, bursitis, tennis elbow and other sports injuries. Also for tonsillitis, herpes, respiratory system infection, candida, thrush and contact dermatitis.

Dose: *If symptoms are acute, take 20-30 drops every hour. If chronic, take 20-40 drops three times a day. Best to pulse (see pages 28 & 49).*

Ingredients: *Fresh Echinacea angustifolia, purpurea root, dried Echinacea angustifolia and pallida roots, fresh Echinacea angustifolia and purpurea flowering herb juice, dried Echinacea purpurea mature seeds.*

Turmeric (*Curcuma longa*, dried rhizome). For inflammation of muscles and synovial membranes of joints in arthritis, myositis and fibromyositis. Useful for gall bladder stones, and inflammation of the gall bladder and liver.

Dose: *Take 10-30 drops three times a day. Best to pulse (see pages 28 & 49).*

Contraindications: *Not in pregnancy.*

Usnea (*Usnea barbata*, dried lichen). Specific for pneumonia, pleurisy, bronchitis, sinusitis, cystitis, urethritis, sore and/or strep throat. Used externally for staph, strep or fungal infection, impetigo, athlete's foot, ringworm or as a douche in Trichomonas infection.

Dose: *Internally: Take 20-40 drops three to five times a day. Best to pulse (see pages 28 & 49). Externally: Use straight or diluted as a wash.*

Uva Ursi (*Arctostaphylos uva-ursi*, dried leaves). For acute cystitis and urethritis accompanied with sharp stabbing-like pain when urinating; kidney or bladder ulceration. For cystitis in paraplegics.

Dose: *Take 20-30 drops four to five times a day for up to* one week to achieve best results. Best to pulse (see pages 28 & 49).

Contraindications: *Not in pregnancy.*

Side effects: *Long term use may irritate the stomach.*

Valerian (*Valeriana officinalis*, fresh Autumn-harvested root). For nervousness, anxiety, and stress-related hypertension. Use for insomnia, emotional depression, poor sleep from pain or trauma, and gastro-intestinal or uterine cramps, especially in the weakened person.

Dose: *Take 20-80 drops as needed. Not for long term use. Best to pulse (see pages 28 & 49).*

Side effects: *Prolonged, continuous use (for over six months) may cause depression.*

Vein Tonic™ (Horse Chestnut/Witch Hazel Complex). Specific for varicose veins, lymphoedema, vascular spasms, chronic circulatory weakness and feeling of heaviness in the legs. Vein Tonic helps prevent cerebrovascular disease and thrombophlebitis. Relieves edema, reduces blood vessel permeability, increases venous and capillary tone and lessens inflammation of blood vessels. Relieves painful cramps in the legs at night and is recommended as a natural substitute for quinine medication.

Dose: *Pulse by taking 25-35 drops twice a day for three weeks. Stop for one week. Repeat.*

Contraindications: *Not in pregnancy.*

Ingredients: *Horse Chestnut, Witch Hazel, Butcher's Broom, Rue, Sweet Clover, Calendula, Milk Thistle, Ocotillo, Oregon Grape root, Stevia.*

California Poppy

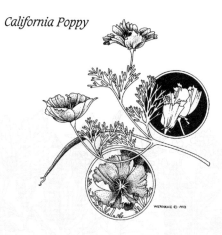

Vitex (*Vitex agnus-castus [Chaste Tree],* dried fruit). For premenstrual syndrome (PMS) caused by excess estrogen or low level of progesterone, menopausal change, and endometriosis. Also for acne and premenstrual herpes on the lips. Stimulates milk production in nursing mothers.

Dose: *Take 15-30 drops as needed. Best results are achieved if taken for a minimum of three to six months.*

Contraindications: *Not in pregnancy. Not while taking oral contraceptives.*

Side effects: *May counteract the effectiveness of birth control pills.*

Wild Cherry Bark (*Prunus serotina*, dried bark). Useful for irritating or chronic cough with excessive expectoration, bronchitis, or whooping cough. Also useful when recuperating from lung or digestive problems, pleurisy, pneumonia or hepatitis.

Dose: *Take 20-60 drops up to four times a day. Best to pulse (see pages 28 & 49).*

Wild American Ginseng (see Ginseng, Wild American)

Wild Oats (See Oat Seeds)

Wild Yam (*Dioscorea villosa*, fresh root). Helps stop cramps or spasms of "hollow organs," such as intestines, gall bladder, uterus, bladder and ureters. Relieves inflammation in acute rheumatoid arthritis, and diverticulosis. Excellent for morning sickness. Helps ease stomach or intestinal irritability after operations.

Dose: *Take 20-40 drops four to five times a day.*

Woodsgrown American Ginseng (see Ginseng, Woodsgrown American)

Yarrow (*Achillea millefolium*, fresh flowering herb). Taken in hot water, causes sweating to assist in easing fever, symptoms of common colds, and amenorrhea

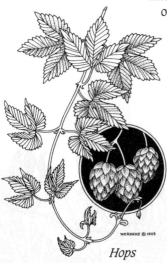

WERNEKE © 1993

Hops

(lack of menstruation). Taken in cold water, eases passive bleeding of the uterus, bladder or lungs; relieves gastric cramps, stomach gas, uterine spasms.

Dose: *Take 15-30 drops every four hours. Best to pulse (see pages 28 & 49).*

Contraindications: *Not in pregnancy.*

Yeast ReLeaf™ (Pau D'Arco/Black Walnut Complex). For intestinal or systemic Candida infection with resulting irregularities: diarrhea or constipation, bloating, low or fluctuating energy levels, vaginitis, menstrual difficulties, and/or very high allergic reactions to foods. Also used for thrush or mouth fungal infection, sinus infection, and certain types of eczema aggravated by Candida. Useful on athlete's foot.

Dose: *Internally: Take 10-25 drops three to four times a day. Best to pulse (see pages 28 & 49). Externally: Use straight, or diluted as a wash.*

Contraindications: *Not in pregnancy.*

Ingredients: *Pau D'Arco, Quassia, Licorice, Echinacea, Myrrh, Yerba Mansa, Black Walnut hulls, Thuja, Astragalus, Garlic.*

Yellow Dock (*Rumex crispus*, dried root). For skin eruptions, acne, eczema, urticaria, psoriasis, accompanied by constipation, jaundice from liver congestion, bad breath and indigestion.

Dose: *Take 20-40 drops twice a day. Best to pulse (see pages 28 & 49).*

Contraindications: *Use cautiously when a history of kidney stones is present.*

Yerba Mansa (*Anemopsis spp.*, dried root). Excellent substitute for Golden Seal. For slow healing conditions such as mouth, gum and throat sores, stomach and duodenal ulcers, colitis, pleurisy and bladder inflammation. Use externally for skin ulcers and boils. Use as a sitz bath for Bartholin gland cysts, perianal fissures and hemorrhoids.

Dose: *Internally: Take 20-40 drops up to four times a day. Best to pulse (see pages 28 & 49). Externally: dilute and apply. Sitz bath: dilute one teaspoon per one quart of water.*

Health Condition Index

This index cross-references recommended herbs for health conditions listed in alphabetical order from A (Abdominal Pain) to Y (Yeast Infection). For detailed explanations of each recommended single herbal extract or formula, consult the **Herbal Repertory** (Chapter 7).

Please note: The herbs recommended for each health condition listed here are the herbs that are most appropriate and useful for that specific condition. For instance, when you read the **Herbal Repertory** (Chapter 7), you will see that several herbs, such as Acnetonic™, Barberry, Chickweed, Dandelion, Echinacea, Gotu Kola, Vitex and Yellow Dock, are indicated in the treatment of acne. All are appropriate but in the interest of helping you choose the most useful herbs, this index limits its recommendations for acne to Acnetonic™, Dandelion, Vitex and Yellow Dock.

As you consult this index, you may also notice that there are specialized conditions such as "Decubitis" listed here that have not appeared previously in this book. Cat's Claw, for instance, is recommended here for Decubitis. But in the **Herbal Repertory** (Chapter 7), Decubitis is not included in the description of Cat's Claw. Cat's Claw is, nevertheless, helpful for that condition. Listing every possible condition under every herb would have made the **Herbal Repertory** (Chapter 7) too lengthy. Therefore, mention of rare or specialized conditions and their recommended herbs is limited to this index. Continue to follow the directions for use of recommended herbs as noted in the **Herbal Repertory** (Chapter 7).

Abdominal pain
Chamomile
Digestonic™
Peppermint
Montezuma's ReLeaf™
Stomach Tonic™

Abcess
Acnetonic™
Dermatonic™
Essiac Tonic™
Golden Seal/Echinacea
    Complex™
Lymphatonic™
Red Root

Abrasions, skin
Calendula
    (externally)
Golden Seal
Lymphatonic™
Propolis

Acne
Acnetonic™
Dandelion
Vitex (around lips)
Yellow Dock (on face
    and shoulders)

**Acquired Immune
Deficiency Syndrome
(AIDS), as support**
Astragalus
Echinacea
Licorice
St. John's Wort
Triple Source
    Echinacea™

Adaptogen
Adrenotonic™

Deep Chi Builder™
Ginsengs (all)
Schisandra
7-Ginsengs™

Addiction
Adrenotonic™
Ginsengs (all)
Oat Seeds

Adrenal
Adrenotonic™
Astragalus
Ginsengs (all)
Licorice

Agitation
Chamomile
Cool Kava Complex™
Deprezac™
Kidalin™
Nervine Tonic™
Skullcap
St. John's Wort

**Aids Related
Complex (ARC)**
Astragalus
Deep Chi Builder™
Echinacea
Licorice
St. John's Wort
Triple Source
    Echinacea™

Alcoholism
Barberry
Kudzu
Liver Tonic™
Milk Thistle

Alertness
Bionic Tonic™
Gingko
Remember Now™

Allergic Rhinitis
Adrenotonic™
Allertonic™
Ephedra (Ma Huang)
Nettle

Allergic Skin Disorders
Allertonic™
Nettle
Schisandra

Allergies, acute
Allertonic™
Ephedra (Ma Huang)
Eyebright
Golden Seal
Nettle

Allergies, prevention of
Adrenotonic™
Allertonic™
Deep Chi Builder™

Altitude Adjustment
Chlorophyll
    Concentrate™

Alzheimer's Disease
Gingko
Gotu Kola
Remember Now™

**Amenorrhea
(lack of menstruation)**
Cycle 1 Estrotonic™
Cycle 2 Progestonic™
Pennyroyal

Amoebic Infection
Barberry
Montezuma's ReLeaf™

Anemia
Alfalfa
Chlorophyll
    Concentrate™
Nettle

Angina
Cardiotonic™
Hawthorn

Antihistamine
Allertonic™
Licorice
Nettle

Anxiety
Chamomile
Cool Kava Complex™
Deprezac™
Kava Kava
Passion Flower
Passion Potion™
Nervine Tonic™
St. John's Wort
Valerian

Appetite, poor
Barberry
Deprezac™
Digestonic™
Gentian

Arrythmia, heart
Cardiotonic™
Hawthorn

Arthritis
Arnica
    (externally)
Arthrotonic™
Cat's Claw
Devil's Claw
Feverfew

Herbaprofen™

Meadowsweet

Asthma, acute

Congest Free™

Decongestonic™

Ephedra (Ma Huang)

Lobelia

Asthma, chronic

Adrenotonic™

Lung Tonic™

Nettle

Passion Flower

Athlete's Foot

Black Walnut Hull
(externally)

Yeast ReLeaf™
(externally)

Usnea
(externally)

Attention Deficit Disorder (ADD)

Kidalin™

Catnip

Chamomile

Attention Deficit Hyperactivity Disorder (ADHD)

Kidalin™

Catnip

Chamomile

Autoimmune Disorders

Adrenotonic™

Deep Chi Builder™

Essiac Tonic™

Ginsengs (all)

7-Ginsengs™

Back Pain

Cran-Bladder ReLeaf™

Herbaprofen™

Kidney Tonic™

PMS ReLeaf™

Valerian

Bacterial Infection

Echinacea

Echinacea/Astragalus
Complex™

Golden Seal/Echinacea
Complex™

Lymphatonic™

Triple Source
Echinacea™

Usnea

Bartholin Gland Cyst

Lymphatonic™

Red Root

Yerba Mansa
(externally)

Bed Sores

Calendula
(externally)

Lymphatonic™

Propolis

Bed Wetting

California Poppy

Horsetail

Bile Secretion

Dandelion

Liver Tonic™

Yellow Dock

Bilirubin, high levels of

Liver Tonic™

Birth Pains, after
- Black Cohosh
- Cramp Bark
- Cramp Releaf™

Bites, bug
- Echinacea, (externally & internally)
- Ivy Itch ReLeaf™ (externally)
- Lymphatonic™ (externally & internally)
- Triple Source Echinacea™ (externally & internally)

Bitter Tonic
- Barberry
- Digestonic™
- Gentian

Bladder Irritation or Infection
- Cran-Bladder ReLeaf™
- Gravel Root
- Kidney Tonic™
- M-Roid ReLeaf™
- Pipsissewa
- Uva Ursi

Bleeding
- Bayberry
- Horsetail
- Red Raspberry
- Shepherd's Purse
- Yarrow

Blepharitis
- Eyebright (externally, diluted)

Bloating
- Catnip
- Digestonic™
- Fennel
- Peppermint
- Stomach Tonic™
- Yeast ReLeaf™

Blood Builder
- Chlorophyll
- Yellow Dock

Blood Cholesterol, high
- Adrenotonic™
- Cholesterotonic™
- Deep Chi Builder™
- Siberian Ginseng
- Seven Ginsengs™
- Wild American Ginseng
- Woodsgrown American Ginseng

Blood Cleanser
- Acnetonic™
- Burdock
- Dandelion
- Dermatonic™
- Liver Tonic™

Blood Poisoning
- Echinacea
- Golden Seal/Echinacea Complex™
- Lymphatonic™
- Triple Source Echinacea™

Blood pressure, high
  HB Pressure Tonic™
  Passion Flower
  Valerian

Blood Sugar, high
  Blueberry

Blood Sugar, low
  Adrenotonic™
  Licorice
  Siberian Ginseng

Blood Triglycerides, high
  Cholesterotonic™
  Siberian Ginseng
  Seven Ginsengs™
  Wild American Ginseng
  Woodsgrown American
    Ginseng

Boils
  Burdock
  Dandelion
  Dermatonic™
  Lymphatonic™
  Yellow Dock

Breasts, sore
  Dong Quai
  Pennyroyal
  PMS ReLeaf™
  Vitex

Bronchioles
  Golden Seal/Echinacea
    Complex™
  Lung Tonic™
  Mullein
  Osha
  Respiratonic™

Bronchitis, acute
  Golden Seal
  Golden Seal/Echinacea
    Complex™
  Osha
  Pleurisy Root
  Respiratonic™
  Usnea

Bronchitis, chronic
  Lung Tonic™
  Mullein
  Wild Cherry Bark

Broncho-spasms
  Adrenotonic™
  Licorice
  Lobelia
  Lung Tonic™
  Osha
  Respiratonic™

Bruise
  Arnica
    (externally)

Burns, skin
  Calendula
    (externally)
  Lymphatonic™

Bursitis
  Arthrotonic™
  Cat's Claw
  Echinacea
  Herbaprofen™
  Triple Source
    Echinacea™

Calcium Absorption
  Alfalfa
  Horsetail
  Nettle

Cancer, prevention of
Deep Chi Builder™
Essiac Tonic™
Red Clover

Cancer, support during treatment
Adrenotonic™
Deep Chi Builder™
Essiac Tonic™
Triple Source Echinacea™

Candidiasis (Candida)
Black Walnut Hull
Cat's Claw
Yeast ReLeaf™

Canker Sores
Bayberry
Digestonic™
Golden Seal
Mouth Tonic™

Car sickness
Ginger

Cat Scratch Disease
Lymphatonic™

Catarrh (mucus)
Golden Seal
Golden Seal/Echinacea Complex™
Hyssop
Osha
Yerba Mansa

Cerebrovascular Disease, prevention of
Deep Chi Builder™
Vein Tonic™

Chemical Exposure
Chaparral
Echinacea
Liver Tonic™

Chest Cold
Elderberry (preventative)
Golden Seal/Echinacea Complex™
Lymphatonic™
Osha
Respiratonic™

Childbirth
Black Cohosh
Blue Cohosh

Cholesterol, elevated
Adrenotonic™
Cholesterotonic™
Deep Chi Builder™
Siberian Ginseng
7-Ginsengs™
Wild American Ginseng
Woodsgrown American Ginseng

Chronic Fatigue Immuno-Deficiency Syndrome (CFIDS)
Adrenotonic™
Essiac Tonic™
Lomatium
Lymphatonic™

Chronic Obstructive Pulmonary Disease (COPD)
Lung Tonic™
Mullein
Osha

Pleurisy Root
Respiratonic™

Circulation
Cayenne
Ginger
Gingko
Vein Tonic™

Cirrhosis
Liver Tonic™
Milk Thistle

Colds, first day
Echinacea
Elderberry
Triple Source
Echinacea™

Colds, prevention of
Deep Chi Builder™
Echinacea
Echinacea/Astragalus
Complex™
Triple Source
Echinacea™

Colds, unshakable
Lymphatonic™
Red Root

Colic
Chamomile
Herbaprofen™
Nervine Tonic™
Peppermint
Stomach Tonic™
Peppermint

Colitis
Cat's Claw
Chamomile
Golden Seal

Peppermint
Stomach Tonic™

Common Cold
Echinacea
Golden Seal/Echinacea
Complex™
Lymphatonic™
Osha
Respiratonic™
Triple Source
Echinacea™

**Common Cold,
prevention of**
Deep Chi Builder™
Echinacea
Echinacea/Astragalus
Complex™
Triple Source
Echinacea™

Concentration
Gingko
Gotu Kola
Remember Now™

Congestion
Allertonic™
Congest Free™
Decongestonic™
Ephedra (Ma Huang)
Respiratonic™

Conjestive Heart Failure
Cardiotonic™
Hawthorn

Conjunctivitis
Allertonic™
Eyebright
(externally, diluted)
Lymphatonic™

Constipation
Barberry
Dandelion
Liver Tonic™
Montezuma's ReLeaf™
Yellow Dock

Contraction, to stimulate uterine
Black Cohosh
Blue Cohosh

Convalescence
Deep Chi Builder™
Ginsengs (all)
Passion Potion™

Coughs
Lobelia
Lung Tonic™
Mullein
Osha
Osha Root Complex Syrup™
Respiratonic™
Singer's Saving Grace™

Cramps, intestinal
Catnip
Chamomile
Herbaprofen™
Peppermint
Stomach Tonic™
Valerian

Cramps, in legs at night
Vein Tonic™

Cramps, menstrual
Black Cohosh
Blue Cohosh
Cramp Bark

Cramp ReLeaf™
Herbaprofen™
Meadowsweet
PMS ReLeaf™

Cuts, slow healing
Deep Chi Builder™
Lymphatonic™
Propolis (externally)

Cystitis
Cran-Bladder ReLeaf™
Damiana
Gravel Root
Kidney Tonic™
Pipsissewa
Uva Ursi

Cysts, breast, ovarian or uterine
Lymphatonic™
Red Root

Cytomegalovirus Infection
Astragalus
Deep Chi Builder™
Echinacea/Astragalus Complex™
Lomatium
Passion Potion™

Dandruff
Burdock
Dermatonic™

Debility
Adrenotonic™
Bionic Tonic™
Deep Chi Tonic™
Ginsengs (all)

Passion Potion™
7-Ginsengs™

Decubitis
Cat's Claw
Chamomile
Lymphatonic™
(internally)
Yerba Mansa

Dentures, sores from
Echinacea
Golden Seal
Mouth Tonic™
Myrrh
Propolis
Yerba Mansa

Deodorizer, intestinal
Chlorophyll
Concentrate™

Depression
Cool Kava Complex™
Damiana
Deprezac™
Ginsengs (Chinese Kirin
Red, Wild American,
Woodsgrown
American)
Passion Potion™
7-Ginsengs™
St. John's Wort

Dermatitis
Burdock
Dandelion
Dermatonic™
Ivy Itch ReLeaf™
Lymphatonic™
Yellow Dock

Diabetes, adult onset
Blueberry
Gingko

Diarrhea
Bayberry
Black Walnut Hull
Golden Seal
Montezuma's ReLeaf™
Propolis
Yeast ReLeaf™
Yerba Mansa

Digestion, poor
Barberry
Digestonic™
Gentian

Diuretic
Chickweed
Dandelion
Kidney Tonic™
Pipsissewa

Diverticulitis
Cat's Claw
Digestonic™
Peppermint

Dizziness
Ginger
Gingko
Remember Now™

Drug therapy, support, during
Adrenotonic™
Alfalfa
Deep Chi Builder™
7-Ginsengs™

Duodenal Ulcers
Barberry
Chamomile   ⇨

Digestonic™
Slippery Elm
Stomach Tonic™

Dysentery
Bayberry
Cat's Claw
Montezuma's ReLeaf™
Para-Free™
Yerba Mansa

Dyspepsia
Chamomile
Peppermint
Stomach Tonic™

Ears
Gingko
Osha
Mullein/Garlic Ear
    Drops™
Remember Now™

**Earache, from
congestion**
Congest Free™
Decongestonic™
Golden Seal/Echinacea
    Complex™
Ephedra (Ma Huang)
Mullein/Garlic Ear
    Drops™
Osha

Ear Infection
Golden Seal/Echinacea
    Complex™
Lymphatonic™
Mullein/Garlic Ear
    Drops™

Eczema
Burdock

Dandelion
Dermatonic™
Ivy Itch ReLeaf™
    (externally)
Nettle
Red Clover

Emphysema
Lung Tonic™
Mullein
Osha
Respiratonic™

Endometriosis
Cycle 2 Progestonic™
Vitex

Endurance, lack of
Adrenotonic™
Astragalus
Deep Chi Builder™
7-Ginsengs™

Energy
Adrenotonic™
Bionic Tonic™
Deep Chi Builder™
Ginsengs (all)

Entamoeba
Black Walnut Hull
Para-Free™

Enteritis
Catnip
Chamomile
Stomach Tonic™

Epstein Barr Virus
Astragalus
Deep Chi Builder™
Echinacea/Astragalus
    Complex™

Lomatium

Estrogen Deficiency
Black Cohosh
Cycle 1 Estrotonic™
Dong Quai

Exhaustion
Adrenotonic™
Deep Chi Builder™
Ginsengs (all)
Oat Seeds
Passion Potion™
7-Ginsengs™

Expectorant
Hyssop
Osha
Osha Root Complex
    Syrup™
Respiratonic™

Extremities, cold
Cayenne
Ginger

Eye
Eyebright
    (externally, diluted
    & internally)

Eyes, mild infection
Eyebright
    (externally, diluted
    & internally)
Golden Seal/Echinacea
    Complex™
Lymphatonic™

Fasting
Alfalfa
Burdock
Dandelion
Lymphatonic™

Fatigue
Adrenotonic™
Astragalus
Bionic Tonic™
Chlorophyll
    Concentrate™
Deep Chi Builder™
Deprezac™
Kava Kava
7-Ginsengs™
Wild American Ginseng
Woodsgrown American
    Ginseng

Fatty Liver
Liver Tonic™
Milk Thistle

Fermentation, intestinal
Digestonic™
Peppermint
Stomach Tonic™

Fertility, low female
Cycle 1 Estrotonic™
Cycle 2 Progestonic™
Dong Quai
Vitex

Fertility, low male
Prostatonic™
Saw Palmetto

Fever
Golden Seal/Echinacea
    Complex™
Meadowsweet
Pennyroyal
Yarrow

**Fibroid cysts, breast,
uterus, ovarian**
Lymphatonic™   ⇨

Red Root
Vitex

Fibromyalgia
Arthrotonic™
Devil's Claw
Herbaprofen™
Meadowsweet
Turmeric

Fibrositis
Arthrotonic™
Devil's Claw
Meadowsweet
Herbaprofen™
Turmeric

Flatulence
Chamomile
Fennel
Hyssop
Peppermint
Stomach Tonic™

Flu
Catnip
Echinacea/Astragalus
  Complex™
Elderberry
Ginger
Golden Seal/Echinacea
  Complex™
Lomatium
Lymphatonic™
Osha
Triple Source
  Echinacea™

**Free Radicals
Scavenger**
Gingko
Remember Now™

Fungal Infection
Black Walnut Hull
Usnea
Yeast ReLeaf™

Gall Bladder
Dandelion
Liver Tonic™
Peppermint
Turmeric
Wild Yam

Gallstones, mild
Herbaprofen™
Liver Tonic™

Gas
Chamomile
Fennel
Hyssop
Peppermint
Stomach Tonic™

Gastric Ulcers
Cat's Claw
Chamomile
Licorice
Stomach Tonic™

Gastritis/Gastro-enteritis
Cat's Claw
Chamomile
Golden Seal
Marshmallow
Meadowsweet
Stomach Tonic™

Giardial Infection
Barberry
Montezuma's ReLeaf™
Para-Free™

Gingivitis
Bayberry
Golden Seal
Mouth Tonic™
Myrrh
Propolis
Yerba Mansa

Gout
Arthrotonic™
Chickweed
Cholesterotonic™
Devil's Claw
Shepherd's Purse

Gums
Bayberry
Golden Seal
Mouth Tonic™
Myrrh
Propolis
Yerba Mansa

Hay Fever
Adrenotonic™
Allertonic™
Congest Free™
Decongestonic™
Ephedra (Ma Huang)
Eyebright
Golden Seal
Nettle

Head Cold
Congest Free™
Decongestonic™
Golden Seal/Echinacea
    Complex™

Headache
Feverfew
Hops
Meadowsweet
Migra Free™

Headache, acute
Feverfew
Migra Free™
PMS ReLeaf™

Headache, chronic
Feverfew
Liver Tonic™
Migra Free™

Hearing Disorders
Gingko
Remember Now™

Heart Support
Cardiotonic™
Hawthorn
Motherwort

Heart Strengthener
Cardiotonic™
Deep Chi Builder™
Hawthorn

Heartburn
Digestonic™
Gentian
Hops
Meadowsweet
Peppermint
Stomach Tonic™

Hemorrhoids
Cat's Claw
Collinsonia
M-Roid ReLeaf™
Shepherd's Purse
Yerba Mansa
    (externally)

Hepatitis
- Deep Chi Builder™
- Liver Tonic™
- Milk Thistle
- Red Clover

Herpes
- Cat's Claw
- Echinacea
- Golden Seal
- Lymphatonic™
- Passion Potion™
- Triple Source Echinacea™
- Mouth Tonic™ (on lips)
- Vitex (on lips)

Hiccough
- Passion Flower
- Stomach Tonic™

High Altitude Sickness
- Astragalus
- Chlorophyll Concentrate™
- Schisandra

High Blood Pressure
- HB Pressure Tonic™
- Passion Flower
- Valerian

High Density Lipo-proteins (HDL)
- Cholesterotonic™

Hives
- Allertonic™
- Ivy Itch ReLeaf™ (externally)
- Nettle

Hoarseness
- Collinsonia
- Osha
- Singer's Saving Grace™

Hormone, imbalance
- Cycle 1 Estrotonic™
- Cycle 2 Progestonic™
- Dong Quai
- PMS ReLeaf™
- Vitex

Hormone, shift
- Cycle 1 Estrotonic™
- Cycle 2 Progestonic™
- Black Cohosh
- Dong Quai
- Menopautonic™
- Vitex
- Wild Yam

Hormone, shift with skin flare up
- Acnetonic™
- Cycle 1 Estrotonic™
- Cycle 2 Progestonic™

Hot Flashes
- Dong Quai
- Menopautonic™
- Motherwort

Human Immuno-deficiency Virus (HIV)
- Deep Chi Builder™
- Echinacea
- Echinacea/Astragalus Complex™
- Lymphatonic™
- St. John's Wort
- Triple Source Echinacea™

Hyperactivity
Catnip
Chamomile
Kidalin™

**Hyperactivity,
in children**
Catnip
Kidalin™

**Hyperglycemia
(high blood sugar)**
Blueberry

**Hypersecretion,
of mucus**
Allertonic™
Congest Free™
Decongestonic™
Golden Seal
Ephedra (Ma Huang)
Nettle

Hypertension
HB Pressure Tonic™
Passion Flower
Valerian

Hypochondria
Adrenotonic™
Deep Chi Builder™
Nervine Tonic™

Hypoglycemia
Adrenotonic™
Licorice
Siberian Ginseng

**Illness,
recuperating from**
Adrenotonic™
Deep Chi Builder™
Ginsengs (all)

Lymphatonic™
7-Ginsengs™

Immune System
Astragalus
Deep Chi Builder™
Echinacea
Echinacea/Astragalus
    Complex™
Lymphatonic™
Triple Source
    Echinacea™

Impetigo
Echinacea
Ivy Itch ReLeaf™
    (externally)
Lymphatonic™
Triple Source
    Echinacea™
Usnea
    (externally and
    internally)

Implantation, egg
Cycle 2 Progestonic™

Impotence
Prostatonic™
Saw Palmetto

Indigestion
Barberry
Chamomile
Digestonic™
Hops
Peppermint
Stomach Tonic™

Infants, colic
Chamomile
Stomach Tonic™

Infection

Echinacea

Echinacea/Astragalus
  Complex™

Lymphatonic™

Osha

Propolis

Triple Source
  Echinacea™

Usnea

Inflammation

Arthrotonic™

Bayberry

Calendula
  (externally)

Devil's Claw

Golden Seal

Herbaprofen™

Licorice

Lymphatonic™

Meadowsweet

Nettle

Insect Bites

Echinacea
  (externally &
  internally)

Ivy Itch ReLeaf™
  (externally)

Lymphatonic™
  (internally)

Triple Source
  Echinacea™
  (externally &
  internally)

Insomnia

California Poppy

Chamomile

Cool Kava Complex™

Deep Sleep™

Hops

Passion Flower

Skullcap

Valerian

Intercourse, painful

Cycle 1 Estrotonic™

Cycle 2 Progestonic™

Menopautonic™

Intercourse, urinary infection after

Cran-Bladder ReLeaf™

Kidney Tonic™

Pipsissewa

Uva Ursi

Interferon, production of

Astragalus

Deep Chi Builder™

Echinacea

Echinacea/Astragalus
  Complex™

Lymphatonic™

Triple Source
  Echinacea™

Intestinal Distress

Bayberry

Fennel

Montezuma's Releaf™

Para-Free™

Intestines

Montezuma's ReLeaf™

M-Roid ReLeaf™

Para-Free™

Peppermint

Slippery Elm

Wild Yam

Irritable Bowel Syndrome
Deep Chi Builder™
Peppermint

Jaundice
Dandelion
Liver Tonic™

Jaw, tense
Herbaprofen™
Nervine Tonic™
Valerian

Joints
Arthrotonic™
Black Cohosh
Devil's Claw
Herbaprofen™
Meadowsweet

Khron's Disease
Cat's Claw
Chamomile
Peppermint

Kidney
Burdock
Chickweed
Dandelion
Kidney Tonic™
Horsetail
Pipsissewa
Uva Ursi

Labor
Black Cohosh
Blue Cohosh

Lactation
Fennel
Red Clover
Red Raspberry
Vitex

Laryngitis
Collinsonia
Myrrh
Osha
Singer's Saving Grace™

Leaky Bowel Syndrome
Cat's Claw
Montezuma's ReLeaf™
Para-Free™
Yeast ReLeaf™

Leukorrhea
Black Walnut Hull
Echinacea
Pau D'Arco
Triple Source Echinacea™
Yeast ReLeaf™

Lichen
Black Walnut Hull
Usnea
Yeast ReLeaf™

Ligaments
Echinacea
Triple Source Echinacea™

Liver
Barberry
Dandelion
Liver Tonic™
Milk Thistle
M-Roid ReLeaf™
Peppermint
Turmeric

Low Density Lipoproteins (LDL)
Cholesterotonic™

Lungs, weak
Deep Chi Builder™
Lung Tonic™

Lungs, congested
Hyssop
Osha
Osha Root Complex
Syrup™
Respiratonic™

Lupus, support
Deep Chi Builder™
Echinacea/Astragalus
Complex™
Lymphatonic™

Lymph Nodes
Echinacea
Lymphatonic™
Red Root
Triple Source
Echinacea™

Lymphoedema
Lymphatonic™
Vein Tonic™

Memory, to improve
Gingko
Gotu Kola
Remember Now™

Menopause
Black Cohosh
Dong Quai
Menopautonic™
Motherwort
Passion Flower
Vitex

Menstrual Cramps
Black Cohosh

Blue Cohosh
Cramp Bark
Cramp ReLeaf™
Ginger
Meadowsweet
Motherwort
PMS ReLeaf™

Menstrual cycle, balancing
Cycle 1 Estrotonic™
Cycle 2 Progestonic™

Menstruation, delayed
Damiana
Pennyroyal

Menstruation, excessive bleeding during
PMS ReLeaf™
Red Raspberry
Shepherd's Purse

Menstruation, general
Chlorophyll
Concentrate™
Cycle 1 Estrotonic™
Cycle 2 Progestonic™
Dong Quai
Vitex

Metabolism, balance
Adrenotonic™
Deep Chi Builder™

Metal Exposure
Chaparral
Liver Tonic™

Middle Ear Infection
Echinacea/Astragalus
Complex™
Golden Seal

Golden Seal/Echinacea
Complex™
Lymphatonic™
Mullein/Garlic Ear
Drops™
Osha

Migraine Headache
Chamomile
Feverfew
Migra Free™
PMS ReLeaf™

Milk Production
Fennel
Red Clover
Red Raspberry
Vitex

**Miscarriage,
prevention of**
Cramp Bark
Cramp ReLeaf™
Wild Yam

Mononucleosis
Milk Thistle
Liver Tonic™
Passion Potion™

Mood Elevator
Cool Kava Complex™
Damiana
Deprezac™
Kava Kava
St. John's Wort

Morning Sickness
Cramp Bark
Cramp ReLeaf™
Ginger
Peppermint

Wild Yam

Motion Sickness
Ginger

Mouth
Bayberry
Golden Seal
Marshmallow
Mouth Tonic™
Propolis

Mucous Membranes
Allertonic™
Bayberry
Ephedra (Ma Huang)
Golden Seal
Golden Seal/Echinacea
Complex™
Nettle

Mucus, excess
Elderberry
Golden Seal
Respiratonic™

Muscles
Arnica
(externally)
Arthrotonic™
Cool Kava Complex™
Herbaprofen™
Meadowsweet
Turmeric

Myositis
Arthrotonic™
Herbaprofen™
Meadowsweet
Turmeric

Nausea
Digestonic™   ⇨

111

Ginger
Peppermint
Stomach Tonic™
Wild Yam

Nephritis
Gravel Root
Kidney Tonic™

Nervousness
Chamomile
Cool Kava Complex™
Hops
Kava Kava
Nervine Tonic™
Oat Seeds
Passion Flower
Valerian

Nervous System, exhaustion
Adrenotonic™
Deep Chi Builder™
Nervine Tonic™
Oat Seeds
Passion Flower™

Nervous System, hyperactivity
Deep Sleep™
Kidalin™
Nervine Tonic™
Passion Flower
Skullcap
Valerian

Neuralgia
Feverfew
Herbaprofen™
Nervine Tonic™
Skullcap
Valerian

Neuritis
Herbaprofen™
Nervine Tonic™
Skullcap
St. John's Wort

Nicotine Withdrawal
Adrenotonic™
Licorice
Lobelia
Oat Seeds
Smoke Free Drops™

Opiate Withdrawal
Adrenotonic™
Oat Seeds

Osteoporosis
Arthrotonic™
Dong Quai
Horsetail

Otitis Media
Echinacea/Astragalus Complex™
Golden Seal/Echinacea Complex™
Lymphatonic™
Mullein/Garlic Ear Drops™
Osha

Ovarian Cyst
Lymphatonic™
Red Root
Vitex

Ovulation, enhancer
Cycle 1 Estrotonic™

Ovaries
Black Cohosh
Cycle 1 Estrotonic™

Cycle 2 Progestonic™
Cramp ReLeaf™
Dong Quai
Vitex

Over-exertion, muscle
Arnica
(externally)
Herbaprofen™
Meadowsweet

Pain
Arthrotonic™
Black Cohosh
Blue Cohosh
Herbaprofen™
Meadowsweet
Nervine Tonic™
Skullcap
Valerian

Palpitations
Cardiotonic™
Hawthorn
Motherwort
Passion Flower

Panic Attack
Cool Kava Complex™
Deprezac™
Kava Kava
PMS ReLeaf™
St. John's Wort

Pancreas
Blueberry
Devil's Claw
Licorice

Parasitic Infection
Barberry
Cat's Claw

Montezuma's ReLeaf™
Para-Free™

Peptic Ulcer
Cat's Claw
Chamomile
Meadowsweet
Stomach Tonic™

Perianal Fissure
Collinsonia
M-Roid ReLeaf™
Yerba Mansa
(externally)

Periodontal Disease
Golden Seal
Mouth Tonic™
Myrrh
Propolis
Yerba Mansa

Pharyngitis
Collinsonia
Golden Seal
Myrrh
Osha
Singer's Saving Grace™
Yerba Mansa

Phlebitis
Arnica
(externally)
Vein Tonic™

Pimples
Acnetonic™
Burdock
Dandelion
Dermatonic™
Lymphatonic™

Pinworms
Black Walnut Hull
Para-Free™

Pleurisy
Osha
Pleurisy Root
Respiratonic™
Usnea

Pneumonia
Lomatium
Osha
Pleurisy Root
Respiratonic™
Usnea

Poison Ivy/Oak
Ivy Itch ReLeaf™
Lymphatonic™
Triple Source
    Echinacea™

**Post Partum
Hemorrhage**
Cramp ReLeaf™
Shepherd's Purse

Pregnancy, support
Cycle 1 Estrotonic™
Cycle 2 Progestonic™
Red Raspberry

Pregnant, to get
Cycle 1 Estrotonic™
Cycle 2 Progestonic™
Dong Quai
Vitex

**Pre-Menstrual
Syndrome (PMS)**
Cycle 1 Estrotonic™
Cycle 2 Progestonic™
Dong Quai

Pennyroyal
PMS ReLeaf™
Red Raspberry
Vitex

**PMS, water
retention from**
Chickweed
Dandelion
Kidney Tonic™
PMS ReLeaf™

Progesterone Deficiency
Cycle 1 Estrotonic™
Cycle 2 Progestonic™
Vitex

Prostatitis
Dong Quai
M-Roid ReLeaf™
Prostatonic™
Sarsaparilla
Saw Palmetto

Protozoal Infection
Black Walnut Hull
Para-Free™
Montezuma's ReLeaf™

Psoriasis
Burdock
Dandelion
Dermatonic™
Liver Tonic™
Pleurisy Root
Red Clover

Psychoactive Herbs
Cool Kava Complex™
Deprezac™
Kava Kava
St. John's Wort

Pyorrhea
Golden Seal
Mouth Tonic™
Myrrh
Propolis
Yerba Mansa

Red Blood Cells, low
Chlorophyll
   Concentrate™

Rejuvenation
Adrenotonic™
Deep Chi Builder™
7 Ginsengs™

Relaxation
Chamomile
Cool Kava Complex™
Kava Kava
Nervine Tonic™

Respiratory System, support
Chlorophyll
   Concentrate™
Deep Chi Builder™
Lung Tonic™
Respiratonic™

Restlessness
Cool Kava Complex™
Deep Sleep™
Hops
Kidalin™
Nervine Tonic™
Skullcap
Valerian

Rheumatic Condition
Arthrotonic™

Cat's Claw
Devil's Claw
Herbaprofen™
Meadowsweet

Rhinitis
Allertonic™
Congest Free™
Decongestonic™
Ephedra (Ma Huang)
Nettle

Ringworm
Black Walnut Hull
Usnea
Yeast Releaf™

Sciatica
Herbaprofen™
Nervine Tonic™
Skullcap
Valerian

Sea Sickness
Ginger

Seasonal Affective Disorder (SAD)
Deprezac

Sedative
California Poppy
Deep Sleep™
Hops
Nervine Tonic™
Valerian

Sexual Energy, to decrease
Hops
Skullcap

Sexual Tonic, for men
Damiana
Deep Chi Builder™
Passion Potion™
Prostatonic™
Sarsaparilla
Saw Palmetto

Sexual Tonic, for women
Cycle 1 Estrotonic™
Deep Chi Builder™
Damiana
Dong Quai
Passion Potion™
Sarsaparilla

Shingles
Herbaprofen™
Nervine Tonic™
Passion Potion™
Skullcap

Silica, source of
Horsetail

Sinusitis
Congest Free™
Decongestonic™
Golden Seal
Golden Seal/Echinacea
    Complex™
Ephedra (Ma Huang)
Nettle
Usnea

Skin
Acnetonic™
Burdock
Calendula
    (externally)
Dandelion
Dermatonic™

Skin, sores
Burdock
Dermatonic™
Echinacea
Lymphatonic™
Yellow Dock

Sleeping, excessive
Adrenotonic™
Deep Chi Builder™
Deprezac™
Oat Seeds
St. John's Wort

Sleeping, problems
California Poppy
Deep Sleep™
Deprezac™
Herbaprofen™
Passion Flower
Skullcap
Valerian

Smoking, withdrawal
Adrenotonic™
Lobelia
Oat Seeds
Smoke Free Drops™

Solvent Exposure
Chaparral
Liver Tonic™
Milk Thistle

Spasms, muscles
Feverfew
Herbaprofen™
Nervine Tonic™
Skullcap

Valerian

Spleen
Lymphatonic™
Red Root

Spotting in Pregnancy, prevention of
Red Raspberry

Sprain
Arnica
(externally)
Herbaprofen™

Staph Infection
Golden Seal/Echinacea
Complex™
Usnea

Steroids, withdrawal or substitute
Adrenotonic™
Licorice
Sarsaparilla

Stimulant
Bionic Tonic™
Chinese Kirin Red
Ginseng

Sting, insects
Echinacea
(externally &
internally)
Ivy Itch ReLeaf™
(externally)
Triple Source
Echinacea™
(internally &
externally)

Stomach
Catnip
Chamomile

Digestonic™
Fennel
Gentian
Hops
Peppermint
Stomach Tonic™

Stones, gall bladder
Liver Tonic™
Turmeric

Stones, kidney
Gravel Root

Strain
Arnica
(externally)
Herbaprofen™

Stress
Adrenotonic™
Cool Kava Complex™
Deep Chi Builder™
Ginsengs (all)
Nervine Tonic™
Oat Seeds
Passion Flower
Schisandra
Valerian

Stroke
Cardiotonic™
Gingko
Hawthorn
Remember Now™

Stye
Echinacea
Eyebright
(externally, diluted)
Lymphatonic™
Triple Source Echinacea

Surgery, recuperating from
- Adrenotonic™
- Deep Chi Builder™
- Ginsengs (all)
- Lymphatonic™

Swelling
- Chamomile (externally)
- Echinacea
- Herbaprofen™
- Lymphatonic™
- Triple Source Echinacea™

Synovial Inflammation
- Arthrotonic™
- Devil's Claw
- Herbaprofen™
- Turmeric

Tachycardia
- Cardiotonic™
- Hawthorn
- Motherwort
- Passion Flower

Tendonitis
- Echinacea
- Herbaprofen™
- Horsetail
- Triple Source Echinacea™

Tennis Elbow
- Echinacea
- Herbaprofen™
- Triple Source Echinacea™

Testosterone
- Dong Quai
- Prostatonic™
- Sarsaparilla
- Saw Palmetto

Throat
- Bayberry
- Collinsonia
- Golden Seal/Echinacea Complex™
- Osha
- Osha Root Complex Syrup™
- Respiratonic™
- Singer's Saving Grace™
- Yerba Mansa

Thrombophlebitis
- Cardiotonic™
- Vein Tonic™

Thrush
- Black Walnut Hull
- Mouth Tonic™
- Pau D'Arco
- Yeast ReLeaf™

Thyroid Gland
- Gotu Kola

Tinnitis
- Gingko
- Remember Now™

Tiredness
- Adrenotonic™
- Astragalus
- Deep Chi Builder™
- Ginsengs (all)
- Passion Potion™
- Schisandra
- 7-Ginsengs™

Tonic, general
Adrenotonic™
Deep Chi Builder™
Ginsengs (all)
7 Ginsengs™

Tonsillitis
Echinacea
Golden Seal
Lymphtonic™
Red Root
Triple Source
Echinacea™

Toothache
Echinacea
Herbaprofen™

Tranquilizer
Cool Kava Complex™
Kava Kava
Nervine Tonic™
Passion Flower
Valerian

Trichomoniasis
Black Walnut Hull
Lymphatonic™
Yeast ReLeaf™

Triglycerides, high
Cholesterotonic™
Siberian Ginseng
7-Ginsengs™
Wild American Ginseng
Woodsgrown American
Ginseng

Tumors
Essiac Tonic™
Deep Chi Builder™

Twitching, muscle
Nervine Tonic™
Skullcap

Ulceration
Chamomile
Golden Seal
Golden Seal/Echinacea
Complex™
Myrrh
Propolis
Yerba Mansa

Ulcers, external and/or internal
Cat's Claw
(externally &
internally)
Chamomile
(externally &
internally)
Licorice
(externally &
internally)
Yerba Mansa
(externally
& internally)

Urethritis
Cran-Bladder
ReLeaf™
Kidney Tonic™
M-Roid ReLeaf™
Pipsissewa
Uva Ursi

Uric Acid, to decrease
Arthrotonic™
Blueberry
Burdock
Devil's Claw
Shepherd's Purse

Urinary Tract Infection (UTI)
Cran-Bladder ReLeaf™
Kidney Tonic™
Pipsissewa
Uva Ursi

Urticaria
Allertonic™
Echinacea
Lymphatonic™
Nettle

Uterine Contraction, weak
Black Cohosh
Blue Cohosh

Uterine Cysts (Fibroids)
Lymphatonic™
Red Root
Vitex

Uterus
Black Cohosh
Cramp Bark
Cramp ReLeaf™
Cycle 1 Estrotonic™
Cycle 2 Progestonic™
Dong Quai
Red Raspberry
Vitex

Vagina
Black Cohosh
Dong Quai
Nettle
Pau D'Arco

Vagina, dry
Black Cohosh
Cycle 1 Estrotonic™

Cycle 2 Progestonic™
Dong Quai
PMS ReLeaf™
Menopautonic™
Motherwort
Vitex

Varicocele
M-Roid ReLeaf™

Varicosities
Calendula
Collinsonia
Vein Tonic™

Vertigo
Ginger
Gingko
Remember Now™

Viral Infection
Echinacea
Echinacea/Astragalus Complex™
Elderberry
Golden Seal/Echinacea Complex™
Lomatium
Lymphatonic™
Osha
St. John's Wort
Triple Source Echinacea™

Vitality, low
Adrenotonic™
Deep Chi Builder™
Ginsengs (all)
7-Ginsengs™

Vomiting
Fennel

Ginger
Peppermint
Stomach Tonic™
Wild Yam

Warts
Black Walnut Hull
Yeast ReLeaf™

Water Retention
Chickweed
Dandelion
Kidney Tonic™
Motherwort
PMS ReLeaf™

Weakness
Adrenotonic™
Astragalus
Chlorophyll
    Concentrate™
Deep Chi Builder™
Ginsengs (all)
7-Ginsengs™

White Blood Cells, low
Echinacea
Echinacea/Astragalus
    Complex™
Lymphatonic™
Myrrh
Triple Source
    Echinacea™

Wound
Echinacea
Golden Seal/Echinacea
    Complex™
Usnea

Yeast Infection
Black Walnut Hull
Echinacea/Astragalus
    Complex™
Pau D'Arco
Yeast ReLeaf™

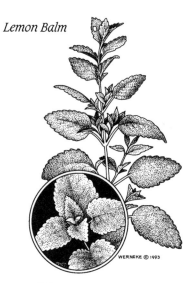

Lemon Balm

WERNEKE © 1993

121

Latin Name—
Common Name Index

Notes on the use of this index:

If you know only the Latin name of an herb, this index will help you find the common name so that you can look it up under its common name in the **Herbal Repertory** (Chapter 7).

Achillea millefolium	YARROW
Althaea officinalis	MARSHMALLOW
Anemopsis spp.	YERBA MANSA
Angelica sinensis	DONG QUAI
Arctostaphylos uva-ursi	UVA URSI
Arnica spp.	ARNICA
Arctium lappa	BURDOCK
Asclepias tuberosa	PLEURISY ROOT
Astragalus membranaceus	ASTRAGALUS
Avena sativa	OAT SEEDS
Berberis vulgaris	BARBERRY
Calendula officinalis	CALENDULA
Capsella bursa-pastoris	SHEPHERD'S PURSE
Capsicum annuum	CAYENNE
Caulophyllum thalictroides	BLUE COHOSH
Ceanothus americanus	RED ROOT
Centella asiatica	GOTU KOLA
Chimaphila umbellata	PIPSISSEWA
Cimicifuga racemosa	BLACK COHOSH
Collinsonia canadensis	COLLINSONIA
Commiphora myrrha	MYRRH
Crataegus spp.	HAWTHORN
Curcuma longa	TURMERIC
Dioscorea villosa	WILD YAM
Echinacea angustifolia	ECHINACEA
Eleutherococcus senticosus	SIBERIAN GINSENG
Ephedra sinica	EPHEDRA (MA HUANG)
Equisetum arvense	HORSETAIL
Eschscholzia californica	CALIFORNIA POPPY
Eupatorium purpureum	GRAVEL ROOT

Tabebuia impetiginosa	PAU D'ARCO
Tanacetum parthenium	FEVERFEW
Taraxacum officinale	DANDELION
Trifolium pratense	RED CLOVER
Turnera spp.	DAMIANA
Ulmus fulva	SLIPPERY ELM
Uncaria tomentosa	CAT'S CLAW
Urtica dioica	NETTLE
Usnea barbata	USNEA
Vaccinium myrtillus	BLUEBERRY
Valeriana officinalis	VALERIAN
Verbascum thapsus	MULLEIN
Viburnum opulus	CRAMP BARK
Vitex agnus-castus	VITEX (CHASTE TREE BERRIES)
Zingiber officinalis	GINGER

The following two herbal extracts do not have Latin names:
CHLOROPHYLL & PROPOLIS

Oats

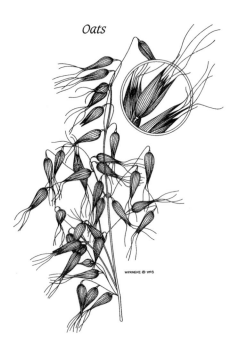

WERNEKE © 1993

124

Suggested Reading

For the lay person:

The following authors present high quality, ethical information that is useful and practical to most everyone. These books can purchased at most natural product stores.

By Daniel Gagnon and Amadea Morningstar

Breathe Free

This book was written because I wanted to share good practical information on how to treat respiratory problems. My frustration with most existing herbal books is that they tell you which herbs to use, but not how much to take and why. Therefore, *Breathe Free* gives you specifics on which foods, supplements and herbs to take. It covers such problems as common colds and flu, hay fever, sore throats, earaches, asthma, pneunomia, bronchitis and emphysema, among other problems.

By Christopher Hobbs

Echinacea, The Immune Herb
Foundation of Health
Ginkgo, Elixir of Youth
Handbook for Herbal Healing
Milk Thistle, The Liver Herb
Natural Liver Therapy
Medicinal Mushrooms
Usnea, The Herbal Antibiotic
Valerian, The Relaxing and Sleep Herb
Vitex, The Women's Herb

Christopher is a good friend of mine. His writing is both scientifically-directed and "user-friendly". His books strike a good balance between imparting high-level scientific research and translating research results into practical information for everyday use.

By David Hoffman

The New Holistic Herbal

The Elder's Herbal

If you were going to buy just one other herbal book for your family (in addition to *Liquid Herbal Drops in Everyday Use*), I would strongly suggest that it be David's *New Holistic Herbal.* Due to its comprehensive approach, I use it as "required reading" for the herbal class that I teach to nursing students.

By Michael Moore

Medicinal Plants of the Desert and Canyon West

Medicinal Plants of the Mountain West

Medicinal Plants of the Pacific West

Michael's great sense of humor turns what could be even the most potentially boring reading into an interesting experience. In his book *Medicinal Plants of the Pacific West,* for instance, his comparison of an herb called Western Skunk Cabbage to the carnivorous plant in the movie *Little Shop of Horrors* is the most humorous review of this herb that I have seen. Michael's incredible knowledge of physiology and profound understanding of the medicinal actions of herbs make his books required reading for anyone who is truly interested in herbal medicine.

By Michael Tierra

The Way of Herbs

Planetary Herbology

The Way of Herbs is a good introduction to herbal medicine. *Planetary Herbology* is a fascinating, eclectic book incorporating points of view from Ayurvedic Medicine, Traditional Chinese Medicine and Western Herbology.

By Susun Weed

Wise Woman Herbal-Healing Wise

Wise Woman Herbal for the Childbearing Years

Wise Woman Herbal for the Menopausal Years

Breast Cancer? Breast Health! The Wise Woman Way

Susun's writings express strong opinions and her books are directed toward empowering women to become involved in their own health care. I highly respect her work and suggest her books to all those interested in expanding their herbal horizons. Susun's poetic side is evident in her work and I really like this aspect of her writing.

Additional reading for the serious student and the health professional:

By Bensky and Gamble
Chinese Herbal Medicine

This is probably the most complete herbal book on the use of Chinese herbs available.

By Finley Ellingwood
American Materia Medica,
Therapeutics and Pharmacognosy

Although first published in 1898, the information in this book is still absolutely relevant.

By Harvey Felter
The Eclectic Materia Medica, Pharmacology
and Therapeutics

Although first published in 1922, information in this book is also still absolutely relevant.

By Michael Moore
See titles listed on page 126.

Michael's understanding of physiology and herbs is so insightful that I also highly recommend his books to those who wish to do an in-depth study of herbal medicine.

By Rudolf Weiss
Herbal Medicine

This book is an excellent source of modern, useful, accurate information presented in a medical framework.

Notes

Echinacea angustifolia